"This is the book that should have been written years ago. It belongs on the shelf of every home, as well as every healthcare practitioner dealing with psychiatric medications. It is practical, up to date, well organized, easy to understand, and immensely useful. This, to me, is a must-have resource for today's mental health."

Daniel A. Hoffman, M.D., Neuropsychiatrist.
Medical Director, Neuro-Therapy Clinic, P.C.
Chief Medical Officer, CNS Response, Inc.

"I'm too pooped to be elegant. But, I'm not going to shut down the computer without saying a quick 'thanks' for what appears to be a fantastic piece of work . . . I HAVE to go to bed, but I could probably stay up just going from one page to the next."

Peter S, Child and Adolescent Psychiatrist

"I just wanted to write to thank you for all the effort you put in to writing your book on psychiatric medicines. I read widely, and your book is beyond doubt the best resource on the subject I have ever come across. Many thanks!"

Bill T, in the UK

"I am now reading your *Medicines for Mental Health* . . . I just wanted to commend you on your exceptional writing skills. What a pleasure to read. Thank you!"

Vicky M

"[Y]ou're awesome . . . You will never know how much your [advice] helped."

Rick W

ii

Medicines for Mental Health

The Ultimate Guide to
Psychiatric Medication

Second Edition

Kevin Thompson, Ph.D.

www.mentalmeds.org

This book is intended to be a useful summary of information regarding treatments for mental illness. Although every effort has been made to provide accurate information, the author and publisher make no warranties that this book is free from error. Nor should the content of this book be construed as medical advice, as it does not recommend any medication, or combination thereof, for any medical problem. The purpose of this book is to provide information for use by patients and physicians in understanding, and selecting, treatments for the patient's illness. Self-medication by patients is not recommended, and the author denies all liability for any damage flowing, directly or indirectly, from actions taken based on information contained herein.

ISBN 1-4196-6954-0
Library of Congress Control Number: 2007903916
Publisher: BookSurge Publishing
North Charleston, South Carolina

Cover design by Kathrine Rend, Rend Graphics & Photography

This book is dedicated to

My wife and daughter, who fill my life with joy and meaning

The many good people, in discussion forums and elsewhere, who have contributed their insight and feedback over the years

The doctors, nurses, therapists, and other healers who dedicate their lives to helping those in need of healing

The scientists, researchers, engineers, and other workers (from the administrative assistants and shipping clerks up through the CEOs and venture capitalists), whose ceaseless labor over decades has made it possible for pharmaceutical companies to provide the medications that we have come to take for granted

Contents

Preface

This book is for people who have a mental illness, or know someone who has a mental illness, and want to know about the types of treatment that are available. If you are one of these people, then read on. You will find more useful information here than you are likely to find anywhere else.

This book is also for medical practitioners and interested laypeople who may not specialize in psychiatric medications, but would like to have a good reference that covers the breadth of available treatments, at a useful depth. If you are a psychologist, therapist, general practioner, nurse, acupuncturist, chiropractor, or anyone else who works with patients who take these medications, you, too, will find more useful information here than you are likely to find anywhere else.

No book of this size can contain all useful information about treatments for mental illness. This is why I have created the companion Web site, *Medicine for Mental Health*, at www.mentalmeds.org. The book packs a great deal of information about how these treatments work, including information on over 100 medications, into a volume of modest size. It does so at the cost of being unable to provide detailed information about every single drug. The Web site picks up where the book leaves off, and provides the highly detailed information about each drug. Together, the book and the Web site accomplish the difficult task of making these medications understandable, providing the details on demand, and opening up an entire world of additional resources to those in need.

Welcome. Welcome to help, and welcome to hope. Welcome to *Medicines for Mental Health*.

Feedback and Advice

I hope you will find this book useful, and I would like to hear your thoughts about improvements. Please send your comments to meds@mentalmeds.org.

I appreciate all messages, but the volume I receive makes it impossible, at times, to reply to every one of them. A more effective way to seek advice is to post questions on public discussion forums over the Internet. Many such forums exist. Here is a brief list of groups that I find informative, and in which I often participate (under the pen-name of Nom dePlume):

alt.support.depression.medication	Medication for depression.
alt.support.depression.manic	Medication and advice for bipolar disorder.
alt.support.schizophrenia	Medication and advice for schizophrenia.

These groups can be found through any standard news reader (Usenet client) program, such as Microsoft's Outlook Express. Alternatively, they may also be found through Google Groups at groups.google.com.

Chapter 1

Introduction

Psychotropic medications affect the functioning of the brain, usually by modifying neurotransmitter chemistry. They are prescribed for a variety of mental illnesses, such as depression, bipolar disorder, anxiety, and schizophrenia.

The number of psychotropic medications is large and growing, so much so that physicians who specialize in the field have difficulty keeping up with developments. In fact, relatively few physicians, even among psychiatrists, can be considered highly knowledgeable in this area, and it is unlikely that any one psychiatrist is well acquainted with all of the available medications. Unfortunately, this is an area where ignorance comes with a cost, in the form of missed opportunities, and dangerous reactions.

The average person who needs medication for a psychiatric disorder is unlikely to know anything about the field, and is often in such a distressed state that research is impossible. Yet the sick person, above all, cares more about the effectiveness and safety of his medication than anyone else.

If the people who care the most about treatment for mental illness know the least, and the people who know the most seldom know enough, then there is a serious need for information on the subject at a level that both the sick and their healers can understand.

This book was written to provide information about the medical treatment of depression, bipolar disorder, schizophrenia, and sexual dysfunction. It was written primarily to assist the sick and suffering in understanding what their medications do, and what their treatment options are. It covers virtually all medications in use at the time of writing, and is organized in a manner that allows the casual reader to skip the technical details, and quickly learn the basics about the medications he needs, or is taking.

At the same time, this book contains enough technical information to be useful for medical practicioners and educated laypeople who wish to understand how these medications work. Nurses and general practitioners, who do not specialize in treating psychiatric disorders, should find it a convenient guide to the available treatments, and a good reference to provide to their patients.

The document is organized by the illness for which the medications are most often prescribed. Each section contains a list of categories of medications and their acronyms. The general properties of each category are described, and a list of individual medications follows. Note that a particular medication, though listed as prescribed for one illness, may be useful and prescribed for others as well.

The remainder of this chapter introduces some basic concepts about how the brain functions, and how mental illnesses are diagnosed and treated. The following chapters focus on specific types of disorder, namely depression, bipolar disorder, schizophrenia, and sexual dysfunction. Chapters and sections may be read (or skipped) in any order, to suit the reader.

Finally, additional information about the medications listed in this book may be found on the author's Web site, at www.mentalmeds.org. The site is designed to be a companion to this book, and it provides detailed prescribing information about each medication, along with additional information and services.

1.1   Sources

Most of the information in this document is generally available from a large number of sources, in which case no specific sources are given. (Specific references are cited for quoted material.) Some resources of particular interest are listed below.

www.crazymeds.org	Quirky, but good medication info and forums
www.driesen.com/index.html	Medication and neurological info
www.pdrhealth.com/index.html	Physician's Desk Reference—very useful
www.nami.org	Self-help, support, and advocacy group
google.fda.gov	US Food and Drug Administration (FDA) Web site
www.mentalhealth.com	Lots of medication information
www.biopsychiatry.com	Odd, but lots of med data, often technical
www.rxmed.com	Good medication database
www.emedicine.com/rc/depression.asp	Good medication database
www.coreynahman.com	Information for the pharmaceutical trade
www.dr-bob.org	Message boards, FAQs, links, and miscellany
www.psycom.net/depression.central.html	Huge site with lots of links
www.needymeds.com	Med suppliers, discount med programs
www.lorenbennett.org/freemeds.htm	Free meds for those with low incomes
home.avvanta.com/~charlatn/depression/tricyclic.faq.html	Good tricyclics info
www.preskorn.com	Good, rather technical information about medications
www.psychopharminfo.com	Current news about medications
www.wholehealthmd.com	Drugs, vitamins, alternative medicine
www.erowid.org/chemicals/maois/maois.shtml	Odd site with MAOI info
www.currentpsychiatry.com/images/pdf/cp0602/CP0602TricyclicTable2.pdf	Reup-

take inhibition

sl.schofield3.home.att.net/medicine/psychiatric_drugs_chart.html	Chemistry
redpoll.pharmacy.ualberta.ca/drugbank	Exhaustive technical medication database
www.drugguide.com	Good database for medications in general
emc.medicines.org.uk	Medications available in the UK

1.2 Answers to Common Questions about this Book

What Do All the Big Words Mean? It is impossible to describe how medications and other treatments work, and what we know about mental illness, without using some terms that are not familiar to most readers. If you do not know what a technical word means, consult the glossary of Chapter 6. The glossary is very complete, and should contain all the definitions you need to understand the main text.

Isn't this Book Obsolete? Yes, it probably is, if it is more than two years old. Medical science progresses rapidly, and new treatments appear every year. Over time, the information in this book will become increasingly incomplete. While it is not possible to update the print in this copy, it is possible to produce new editions that contain the new information.

The newest edition will always be available from www.mentalmeds.org, so look there for updates. The best way to keep up to date is to visit the site, and register to be notified when a new edition is available.

Don't You Need a Medical Degree to Write about Medicine? No. A medical degree (M.D.) provides assurance that a physician is competent to treat his patient's common health problems. By itself, it does not turn a physician into a scientist (few medical doctors perform medical research), nor does it guarantee a deep knowledge of psychotropic medications (few medical doctors specialize in this area, and even among psychiatrists, few perform research).

What is necessary to write a book like this is a basic understanding of brain chemistry, and how medications affect it. This information is readily available for anyone who knows where to look, but is not easy for most people to understand. However, it is comprehensible to anyone with a background in physical science who takes the time to study the subject.

In short, all that is necessary to write a useful book about medicine is an understanding of the subject.

1.3   The Chemicals at the Heart of the Brain

Neurotransmitters are chemicals that are used by neurons (brain cells, or cells in the nervous system) to send signals to each other. A neuron emits a pulse (a "squirt") of a particular neurotransmitter from a vesicle (storage chamber) into the synapse, or synaptic gap, between it and an adjacent neuron. The receptors on the receiving neuron detect the sudden increase in concentration of the emitted neurotransmitter when molecules of the latter "bind," or attach, to them.

If the number of receptors on the receiving neuron that register the increase in neurotransmitter concentration exceeds a threshold, the neuron registers a signal, and takes some action in response (which typically involves sending a signal of its own to its neighbors); otherwise, the neuron ignores the change in neurotransmitter concentration.

Once the concentration of emitted neurotransmitter molecules has exceeded the receving neuron's detection threshold, the neurotransmitter molecules must be removed from the synapse in order to allow for a subsequent signal. Otherwise, the receiving neuron's receptors would quickly be saturated, and cease to function.

The sending neuron has a "reuptake system," a mechanism to absorb the emitted neurotransmitter molecules. Some of the emitted molecules are sucked back in to storage vesicles for re-use, while others are metabolized (destroyed) by the Monoamine Oxidase enzymes. These two mechanisms (reuptake into storage, and metabolization) clear the emitted neurotransmitter molecules from the synapse and prepare it for the next signal.

There are many different types of receptors, and many (over one hundred) known neurotransmitters. The plethora of neurotransmitter and receptor types leads to extremely complex behavior in the brain.

Neurotransmitters commonly affected by psychotropic medications include serotonin, norepinephrine, dopamine, and GABA (gamma-aminobutyric acid). The sequence of chemical reactions involving neurotransmitters is complex and interconnected; as a result, medications that directly affect the chemistry of one neurotransmitter (say, serotonin) do not affect it alone, but others as well. Thus it is a mistake to assume that taking a medication that increases serotonin concentration has no effect on other neurotransmitters, because, in general, it does.

The complexity of brain chemistry, and the complexity of subjective human experience, make it impossible to identify a straightforward connection between a specific neurotransmitter and a particular emotional state, or a particular emotional problem. Nevertheless, some trends can be identified, and are discussed below. (Just bear in mind that all statements about what a particular neurotransmitter does are incomplete, and very rough approximations.)

1.3.1   Dopamine

Dopamine is typically identified as the neurotransmitter most directly associated with pleasure. "Pleasure" includes emotions such as joy, and more physically-oriented sensations such as sensuality, libido, and sexual pleasure. Problems involving dopamine chemistry may reduce or eliminate the capacities for pleasure and libido (sexual desire). People who suffer from an inability to have pleasant feelings (as opposed to having too much in the way of unpleasant feelings) are particularly likely to benefit from increases in dopamine concentration.

Medications (such as amphetamines) that raise dopamine levels often increase energy level as well. This makes sense, as dopamine is a precursor to norepinephrine. Any increase in dopamine concentration can be expected to cause an increase in norepinephrine concentration as well.

1.3.2   Gamma-Aminobutyric Acid (GABA)

GABA, discovered in the 1950s, is a "message-altering" neurotransmitter. It is the major inhibitory neurotransmitter in the central nervous system, and regulates the transmission of signals in the brain.

Neurons receive signals from other neurons in the form of "squirts," or pulses, of neurotransmitters. If a neuron's receptors receive a sufficiently large pulse of neurotransmitters, it registers this pulse as a signal, to be acted on. The neuron's action will very often involve forwarding that signal to adjacent neurons in the same fashion.

The higher the GABA concentration, the less often neurons forward signals to other neurons. Thus GABA has a dampening effect on neural-signal propagation. Too much GABA retards propagation, while too little allows too much propagation. It seems likely that an insufficiency of GABA results in too much signal propagation, which in turn leads to seizures and mania. (See Section 3.2 for more information.)

1.3.3   Glutamate

Glutamate is the most common neurotransmitter in the brain. It's function is roughly the opposite of GABA's, in that it is an excitatory neurotransmitter. The higher the glutamate concentration, the greater the sensitivity of neurons to signals conveyed by other neurotransmitters.

1.3.4   Norepinephrine

Norepinephrine is typically identified as a neurotransmitter most directly associated with energy, meaning the feeling of vigor, and capacity for physical labor. It is also associated with the ability to concentrate. Problems involving norephinephrine chemistry may impair the ability to concentrate, and sap one's energy, leading to fatigue that can become life-threatening if severe enough.

Norepinephrine concentration can be increased by changing how norepinephrine is processed, or by increasing the concentration of dopamine, as dopamine is a precursor to norepinephrine (or, equivalently, norepinephrine is a metabolite of dopamine).

Given the link between norepinephrine and the ability to concentrate, it is not surprising that treatments for Attention Deficity-Hyperactivity Disorder boost norepinephrine levels.

1.3.5   Serotonin

Serotonin is typically identified as the neurotransmitter most directly associated with calmness and general feelings of well-being. Problems involving serotonin chemistry may cause severe emotional disturbance, such as dramatic over-sensitivity to disappointment, extreme melancholia (sadness, e.g., characterized by crying spells), and feelings of worthlessness. Medications that raise serotonin levels often alleviate these symptoms. Unfortunately, increases in serotonin concentration tend to impair libido and sexual function, an effect for which SSRI medications are notorious (though one not limited to them). However, strategies do exist to alleviate these serotonin-induced impairments, for those who require serotonin enhancement to treat their depression.

1.4   The Bad Things that Happen with Good Medications

Few things are as dismaying as taking medication for a mental illness and discovering that you are getting worse, rather than better. There are a variety of reasons why medicines can produce unpleasant results, the most common being that the medication isn't appropriate for the condition. Unfortunately, it is not possible to know in advance which medication will work for a particular person, because individual responses vary so widely. Thus doctors, and patients, must put up with a certain amount of trial and error before finding the right medication. Unfortunately, and by definition, the "wrong" medications will either have no effect, or produce unpleasant effects. This is simply one of the facts of life in the treatment of mental illness as it is today. The wise patient will realize that a degree of patience and stoicism is appropriate when seeking medical treatment.

The following sections describe some of the ways in which medications can cause trouble. The bad news is that there are many opportunities for problems. The good news is that the problems can usually be resolved.

1.4.1   Side Effects and Withdrawal Effects

All medications have the potential for unwanted, unpleasant, or dangerous side effects. This is true whether the medications are prescription drugs, over-the-counter drugs, or herbal products (such as St. John's Wort). Unfortunately, in the case of psychotropic medications, the potential for unwanted side effects approaches certainty. Antidepressant medications that increase serotonin concentration, for example (such as Prozac), are almost guaranteed to suppress libido and sexual function in men and women to some extent. (Methods for alleviating sexual dysfunction are discussed in Section 5.)

The challenge for the physician and patient is to find the medications that provide the greatest benefit with the least negative impact due to side effects. Some people are fortunate, and find medications that completely eliminate their symptoms while having no negative effects. A small number are very unfortunate, and find little or no benefit from existing medications, while experiencing highly unpleasant or even fatal reactions to them. Most are in the middle somewhere, finding substantial benefits while having to find ways to alleviate some degree of side effects.

While the side effects of psychotropic medications are unwanted and occasionally quite unpleasant, they are often transient, disappearing within a couple of weeks of starting the medication. If the effects continue, and are sufficiently unpleasant (or the medication isn't working), the patient will usually stop the medication and try a different one. (Note: Never stop taking one of these medications without consulting with your physician first! Read on to see why this is important.)

Unfortunately, new and unpleasant effects, called withdrawal effects, may appear when a medication is stopped. The good news is that withdrawal effects fade away in time. "In time" may be a few days, a few weeks, or, less commonly, a few months. Some medications generally produce negligible withdrawal effects, while others may produce dramatically unpleasant effects. Withdrawal effects are similar to the benefits of the medication in that they vary widely from person to person, as well as from medication to medication. It is very important to discuss how to stop a medication with your doctor before doing so, as some medications require a careful tapering process (i.e., gradual reduction in dose) in order to avoid unpleasant or dangerous effects.

There are exceptions to the rule that side- and withdrawal effects are temporary. In some cases, they can be permanent, or cause physical damage. As is the case with many drugs, some patients may have drastic reactions to a psychotropic medication (such as liver damage) that may not go away when the medication is stopped. Thus it is always wise to discuss possible dangerous reactions with your physician before trying a medication, and take careful note of any side effects that may foreshadow serious complications. In the case of drugs known to cause liver damage in some people (one of the most common serious dangers for all medications, psychotropic and otherwise), the physician may order routine blood tests to check liver function and detect incipient problems before they become serious.

Medications for psychosis (anti-psychotic, or neuroleptic, drugs) are a special category and have special risks. These medications can cause serious, sometimes permanent, and even fatal conditions called Tardive Dyskinesia and Neuroleptic Malignant Syndrome. For these reasons, the use of anti-psychotic medications must be carefully controlled, and the potentially serious risks weighed against the possible benefits. For some people, the decision may come down to a choice between Tardive Dyskinesia or psychosis, a decidedly unfortunate choice. These problems are a major factor in the drive to find safer medications for the treatment of psychosis, an effort which has produced safer drugs, if not yet as safe as one would wish.

1.4.2   When Antidepressants Drive You Crazy

That psychotropic medications may have undesirable physical side effects is not in dispute, but the extent to which they may have undesirable mental (cognitive or emotional) side effects is a murkier subject. Some such effects are discussed below.

1.4.2.1   Mania

There is one situation in which an antidepressant can almost literally "drive you crazy." Serotonergic medications (such as the SSRI, SNRI, and MAOIs) can trigger manic states in people who have Bipolar Disorder (see Chapter 3). This is a counter-intuitive result, but a well-established one. Thus it is very important to monitor the reaction to these medications for signs of mania. If mania does occur, the patient will require treatment for Bipolar Disorder, not for depression alone.

1.4.2.2   Suicide

The question as to whether antidepressants increase the risk of suicide, especially among teenagers, has been hotly debated. There is some evidence that the rate of attempted suicide among teenagers who take antidepressants is higher than among their peers who do not, but it is not clear whether the difference is due to downswings in mood caused by the medication, or if the medication sometimes improves energy before mood, so that some depressed but energized teens find their suicidal impulses unimpaired by lethargy.

Most depressed teenagers who take an antidepressant are not likely to attempt suicide as a result. However, anyone who is being treated for depression, whether teenaged or not, should be monitored for suicidal tendencies as a matter of course, given that depression by itself is the major cause for suicide. Monitoring for suicidal tendencies should be a standard element of any treatment program, whether medication is involved or not.

1.4.2.3   Anxiety

The neurotransmitter norepinephrine is associated with heightened arousal. At normal levels, it provides an appropriate degree of energy and ability to concentrate. At high levels, it can cause feelings of panic and dread, and physical responses such as elevated heart rate and blood pressure. Elevated levels of norepinephrine are appropriate for "fight or flight" reactions to threats, but not for daily living.

Some people are prone to frequent, even constant, feelings of anxiety. For these people, taking a medication that increases norepinephrine may trigger or worsen these feelings. Thus those who suffer from anxiety disorders should generally avoid noradrenergic medications such as the SNRI, NRI NDRI, and MAOI categories.

1.4.2.4 Emotional Flattening

Serotonergic antidepressants (such as the SSRIs) sometimes "flatten" emotional responses to the point where one feels numb and unresponsive to external events, interactions with people, and so forth. Similarly, medications that blockade (inhibit) dopamine (i.e., the antipsychotics) can suppress the ability to feel pleasure (a condition called "anhedonia"), removing the joy from life.

In the case of serotonergic antidepressants, simply switching to a different medication in the same category often suffices to fix the problem. Unfortunately, the anhedonic response to antipsychotic medications is generally more difficult to address via medication or dose changes, and sometimes cannot be resolved.

1.5 Important: Hormones and Endocrine Disorders

If you have been suffering from fatigue and listlessness, and generally feeling down, you may be able to stop after reading this section. You may be suffering from an endocrine (hormonal) disorder, rather than depression *per se.*

An endocrine disorder is any health problem that arises from having too little, or too much, of any hormone. (Problems with the thyroid hormones, triiodothyronine, or T3, and levothyroxine, or T4, are particularly common.) Typical endocrine problems include

Hyperthyroidism. High levels of thyroid hormones. Hyperthyroidism causes many problems, including weight loss, extreme appetite, weakness, loss of libido, apathy, irritability, depression, and other symptoms.

Hypothyroidism. Low levels of thyroid hormones. Hypothyroidism causes many problems, including fatigue, impaired memory and alertness, difficulty thinking, slowed metabolism, weight gain, loss of libido, anxiety, depression, and other symptoms.

Hashimoto's thyroiditis. An autoimmune disease, in which the body's immune system produces antibodies that attack the cells of the thyroid gland. This illness causes hypothyroidism, and all the symptoms of hypothyroidism, along with swelling and pain in the thyroid gland (in the neck), and flu-like symptoms that are characteristic of autoimmune diseases.

Hypogonadism. Low levels of reproductive hormones, namely testosterone in men, and estradiol and progesterone in women (although women can suffer from too-low levels of testerone as well, which can impair libido). Symptoms of hypogonadism include loss of energy and libido, fatigue, deterioration of mental faculties, and depression.

Hyperprolactinemia. High levels of prolactin. Symptoms of hyperprolactinemia include loss of libido, sexual dysfunction, and depression, in both men and women. Women may suffer from menstrual problems, infertility, hirsutism, or obesity. Sperm production in men may be reduced or absent.

Hypopituitarism. Low levels of hormones produced by the pituitary gland: prolactin, somatropin (growth hormone, or GH), luteinizing hormone (LH), follicle stimulate hormone (FSH), thyroid stimulating hormone (TSH), and adrenocorticotropic hormone (ACTH). Low levels of somatropin and TSH can produce marked energy loss, and deterioration of mood and mental function, similar to hypothyroidism.

The above list is not exhaustive, as many other endocrine disorders exist, but it does capture some of the more common ones that can produce depression symptoms.

As endocrine disorders can cause many of the symptoms of emotional illness, it is important to have a thorough checkout of possible hormonal problems before concluding that the problem is in the brain, rather than the endocrine system. Antidepressant medication will not solve hormonal problems! Fortunately, most common endocrine problems (other than diabetes) can be treated easily. Discuss the possibility of endocrine problems with your doctor. (If possible, seen an Endocrinologist, rather than a General Practitioner or family doctor, for this purpose.)

1.6   Diagnosis and Treatment of Mental Illness

The classic approach to treating mental illness is the same as for treating any illness: First, diagnose the illness, and second, prescribe a type of treatment (medication or otherwise) known to be effective for treating that illness.

Unfortunately, treating mental illness is more difficult than treating a physical illness, such as a bacterial infection, for two reasons: We do not understand the mechanism of the illness, and we lack objective tests useful in the diagnosis and treatment of the illness.

The mechanism problem is a serious one, which affects the treatment process from beginning to end. Because we do not know what causes the various mental illnesses, we cannot even identify them by their cause, but only by their symptoms. A diagnosis such as Major Depressive Disorder is simply a name for a list of symptoms. It is quite possible that such a diagnosis applies to several different illnesses, which operate by different mechanisms, but produce similar symptoms. Thus a medication that, by chance, happens to work well for one of the unidentified illnesses, may not work at all for another. The result is that the medication is described as having a success reate of, say 30%, in treating Major Depressive Disorder, while in fact it works at close to 100% for one of the illnesses, and not at all for the others.

Another problem that stems from a lack of understanding of the mechanism of mental illness is that it is impossible to design a treatment for an illness when one does not know what the illness does. Thus the current treatments for mental illnesses represent many years of trial and error, rather than targeted design. When a medication is discovered that has some benefits, researchers study its effects, and experiment with medications that have similar, but not identical, mechanisms. This type of experimentation helps not only to identify better medications, but to uncover some information about the mechanisms that are involved in the illness. This type of experimentation is responsible for much of our understanding of mental illness, such as it is.

The lack of objective tests is another serious problem. Physicians diagnose mental illness based on the evidence. However, physical illnesses produce not only subjective symptoms (i.e., how the patient feels), but also objective indications that can be observed and measured (e.g., fever, swelling, and bacteria that can be cultured and identified). In contrast, physicians have had to rely entirely on subjective symptoms to diagnose mental illness. Once again, the subjective reports of symptoms cannot reliably distinguish between cases of mental illness with similar symptoms but different origina, and provide a decidely imperfect guide to useful diagnosis.

The limitations on current abilities to diagnose and treat mental illness should not be disheartening. Psychiatry has come a very long way in the last fifty years, and medical treatment of mental illness will continue to improve. Even now, millions of people find relief from the crushing burden of mental illnesses that would have doomed them to misery and early death only fifty years ago. The majority of people who seek treatment for depression and bipolar disorder do so successfully, provided they are willing to invest the time and effort required to find the best medications for them. Even schizophrenia has yielded, albeit imperfectly, to the advance of medical science.

Over time, scientific research will cast more and more light onto the functioning of the brain, and onto the causes and treatment of mental illness.

1.7 Standard Treatments for Mental Illness

Few types of treatment work for a wide variety of mental illnesses. Most are specific to particular illnesses, such as depression, bipolar disorder, and schizophrenia. A few, however, are broadly applicable across multiple types of illness, and are discussed here.

1.7.1 Therapy

Therapeutic approaches may be useful in situations where the depression arises solely from behavioral or situational factors that can be improved by changes in thought patterns and behavior. Therapy may also be useful in conjunction with medical treatment, especially when adjustment to an improved mood presents new challenges to the individual. Therapy, especially cognitive-behavioral therapy (which focuses on improving thought patterns and behavior), is often recommended in conjunction with medication.

The range of available therapies is almost limitless. Examples of different schools of therapy include psychoanalysis, psychodynamic therapy, Jungian therapy, cognitive behavioral therapy (CBT), gestalt therapy, humanistic therapy, dialectical behavior therapy (DBT), rational emotive therapy, exposure therapy, interpersonal therapy, play therapy, and so on. There are also a variety of techniques that can be used to bring about specific results within the context of therapy, such as neuro-linguistic programming (NLP), hypnotherapy, and eye movement desensitization reprocessing (EMDR).

In practice, most therapists draw on several schools of therapy, blending approaches to suit their own preferences and their patients' needs. This approach is an eclectic one, and is often referred to as *eclectic therapy*.

There are really just a few things one should know about therapy as an approach to treating mental illness.

- The best predictor of success in therapy is the rapport, or quality of the relationship, between the therapist and patient. It is important to find a therapist with whom you can have a good working relationship.[1] Keep this fact in mind when you interview therapists, and be prepared to interview several until you find one you like.

- Therapy can be useful for people with depression, bipolar disorder, and schizophrenia, but while some (not all) cases of depression can be resolved through therapy alone, medication is normally required to treat bipolar disorder and schizophrenia. Bipolar disorder and schizophrenia are believed to arise from neurological abnormalities; while they may be worsened by stress of various kinds, they cannot be resolved solely by addressing factors that cause stress. Depression, on the other hand, can sometimes arise entirely as a response to stress, and fade away as the stressful problems are resolved. More often, though, it appears to arise from a combination of neurological factors and external factors (life situation and relationships). Medication can address the former, but not the latter. For these reasons, depression is more likely to be resolved by a combination of therapy and medication.

---

[1] Why "working relationship?" Because the purpose of therapy is to work on improving your life. The therapeutic relationship may be a friendly one, but the therapist is not there to be your friend. He is there to help you work out your problems.

1.7.2 Electro-Convulsive Therapy (ECT)

Electroconvulsive Therapy (ECT) is an electrical-stimulation technique used to treat severe depression, bipolar disorder, schizophrenia and psychosis, and catatonia. It is a remarkable fact that ECT is an effective treatment for so many apparently unrelated types of mental illness. It is perhaps equally remarkable that so little is known about why it works, beyond the consensus that it is the seizure induced by ECT that leads to the benefits.

During an ECT session, the patient is given a general anesthetic to induce brief unconsciousness, and then a voltage is applied to cause an electric current to flow through one (right lateral) or both (bilateral) sides of the brain, inducing a seizure. For reasons that are not well understood, this electrically-induced seizure can dramatically alleviate depression.

Bilateral treament acts more rapidly than unilateral treatment, but has more severe side effects. Right unilateral treatment produces less severe memory loss, and is preferred for depression. Bilateral treatment is generally restricted to emergency situations involving severe depression with psychosis, severe manic episodes, severe psychotic episodes, and catatonia.

ECT is typically used in these circumstances:

1. When it is essential to provide the fastest-possible relief for depression, mania, or psychosis (for example, in the case of someone who is suicidal).

2. When medications have proven ineffective, and symptoms remain severe.

3. For patients with bipolar disorder who need immediate stabilization of their condition, or who are experiencing severe manic episodes. ECT helps both the manic and depressive aspects of this disorder, something that is not normally true for individual medications.

4. For patients with catatonia, a dangerous condition that is often resistant to medication.

ECT is a proven technique. It does not always work, but it works more often than medication for severe depression, and generally as well as medications for bipolar disorder and schizophrenia. It often is the only treatment that works for catatonia.

There are a number of drawbacks to ECT, including

- **Practical Difficulties.** Access to ECT may be difficult, as it is not a common treatment. Also, the expense, and the overhead in terms of time and care that the treatment entails, make it burdensome.

- **Short-term memory loss.** ECT typically causes short-term memory loss, and possibly some temporary impairment of ability to think clearly.

- **Possible long-term deficits.** There are many anecdotal accounts of long-term, even permanent, impairment of memory, ability to think, and ability to experience the normal range of human emotion. These claims have not been confirmed by clinical studies to date. Those who assert the truth of these claims explain this discrepancy by saying that the studies do not measure these types of deficits. As of this writing, no conclusive evidence exists to settle the debate.

It should also be said that some people not only respond well to ECT, but do so without experiencing significant deficits. For these people, most of whom have exhausted the set of available medications, ECT is very much a life saver.

These drawbacks, plus a somewhat sensational and checkered history of past abuse, has led physicians and possible candidates to shy away from ECT. However, ECT should be considered for the circumstances described above.

1.7.3   Medication

While no one medication is effective at treating all types of mental illness, the general strategy of medication applies to more types of mental illness than any other.[2] Medication has eclipsed all other forms of treatment for mental illness by any measure. The success of medication as a strategy is very much a function of its effectiveness, its accessibility, and its relatively low cost compared to the alternatives (where alternatives exist, which is not always the case).

The combination of effectiveness and cost-effectiveness has resulted in a steady migration towards medication, and a steady erosion of access to alternatives (such as therapy and ECT). This trend is particularly evident when one considers that health insurance plans typically pay for medications without limit, but place caps on payments for therapy.

Further details about the use of medication in treating mental illness may be found in the following chapters, as the subject is the main focus of this book. However, the focus on medication should not mislead the reader into thinking that other strategies are without value, when, in fact, they may have great value. What matters in the end is not the path to success, but its achievement. The ultimate criterion for judging treatments of mental illness is effectiveness. The best strategy is always the one that gives the best results.

1.8   Looking to the Future

For the most part, this text focuses on standard medical treatments for mental illness, meaning treatments that have been approved by the US Food and Drug Administration, better known as the FDA. However, the state of the art in medical

---

[2]This does not mean that all forms of mental illness can be treated by medication, but that more can be treated by medication than by any other approach.

treatment outpaces the imprimatur of the FDA, as anecdotal evidence accumulates regarding new and effective uses of existing prescription medications. It is for this reason that known uses of these medications is divided into FDA-approved *on-label* and unapproved *off-label* uses throughout.

All existing treatments for mental illness have limitations. These limitations are felt most painfully by those whom they do not help, or for whom they are too expensive, or simply unavailable. Thus it is worth considering some of the novel treatment methods which are becoming available. These methods are not well known, and are not widely accepted by the medical community. However, lack of wide acceptance is typical for new treatments, and by itself says nothing about their usefulness.

Some of these new treatments are described in the following sections. They must be regarded as experimental at this point, and their appearance in this text should not be taken as an endorsement. How well these treatments work remains to be seen, but the effort to generate new paradigms for the treatment of mental illness should be applauded.

1.8.1   Correlation Methods

The standard paradigm of "diagnose and treat" relies strongly on the concept of diagnosis as an organizing principle, around which the conceptual framework of illness and treatment is constructed. It is worth keeping in mind that the notion of diagnosis is a human concept, not a natural phenomenon. Likewise, diagnosis is important to the patient primarily as a stepping stone on the way to recovery, not as something of value in itself (though it should be said that much comfort can indeed come from knowing what to expect of an illness, which is part of what follows from a diagnosis).

The concept of diagnosis may not be nearly as useful for mental illness as for physical illness. It may be that the underlying mechanisms of both illness and its treatment are so varied, with no firm boundaries between disorders at the level of mechanism, that diagnostic categories will ultimately prove less useful than alternative paradigms for organizing information.

One alternative to the classic paradigm of "diagnose and treat" is a new one, which might be described as "correlate and treat." *Correlation methods* either reduce the significance of diagnosis, or omit the diagnostic stage entirely, and instead focus on the statistical correlation between quantitative measurements, treatments, and outcome.

The novel aspects of the correlation paradigm are

1. The introduction of quantitative measurements for use in treating mental illness

2. Reliance on correlation between measurement, outcome, and treatment type

3. The deprecation or elimination of diagnosis as a requirement for treatment

1.8.1.1   The Referenced EEG Method (rEEG)

The Referenced EEG method (rEEG) is an approach developed by a company named CNS Response (www.cnsresponse.com). It is based on the premise that mental illnesses are associated with abnormal brain activity, and that the abnormal brain activity produces measurable deviations from the norm in electroencephalogram (EEG) recordings. The company maintains a database of normal and abnormal EEG measurements, as well as EEG measurements for people who have taken psychotropic medications of different kinds.

Statistical analysis is then used to predict how an individual with a particular set of abnormal measurements will respond to the medications in the database. Medications are ranked by effectiveness at restoring normal activity. The result of the process is a recommendation for one or more medications predicted to be most effective for the patient.

1.8.1.2   Neurotransmitter Assessment

The premise behind neurotransmitter assessment is that it is possible to measure neurotransmitter levels for an individual to a useful degree of accuracy, to identify deficiencies or excesses of neurotranmsitters, and to restore the proper levels of neurotransmitters through the use of the appropriate chemicals.

While "appropriate chemicals" could include both prescription and non-prescription substances, a company named NeuroScience, Inc. currently recommends non-prescription amino-acid supplements. NeuroScience (www.neurorelief.com) measures neurotransmitter and hormone concentrations in saliva, urine, or blood, and analyzes deviations from the norm. The company then identifies a set of amino-acid supplements whose purpose is to restore concentrations of neurotransmitters and hormones to normal levels.

1.8.1.3   Comparison of rEEG and Neurotransmitter Assessment

It is impossible to compare the effectiveness of these two techniques, as the necessary studies have not been done. However, one can compare and contrast them in terms of science and philosophy.

CNS Response uses a standard diagnostic tool, the EEG, in a new way. The rEEG correlation method tries to identify the best medications to treat an illness. The means by which the identification is made is novel, as is the use of any quantitative measurement in psychiatry, but the philosophy of ordering a laboratory test and then prescribing medication is very much in the mainstream of standard medical practice. It requires no stretch of the imagination to picture psychiatrists ordering this type of test routinely in a few years, much as an endocrinologist would order tests for hormone levels.

The hurdles to be overcome for the rEEG correlation method include acquiring the imprimatur of successful clinical tests, and the culture change (specific to psychiatry) of never ordering lab tests because none have ever been available.

NeuroScience, Inc. uses classic chemical-assay techniques on standard types of laboratory samples (urine, saliva, and blood). It is true that the specific measurements made are not standard, and their use in identifying neurotransmitter problems is new, but where the company most clearly departs from standard medical practice is in recommending amino-acid supplements instead of prescription medications.

This strategy bypasses the bottleneck of traditionally conservative physicians, and the burdensome requirements for FDA approval. The tests and supplements can be supplied by any type of healthcare practitioner, as neither requires a doctor to write a prescription.[3]

The hurdles to be overcome for the neurotransmitter-assessment method include market acceptance by non-physician healthcare practitioners and their patients, and avoidance of regulatory intervention by the FDA. Should the company decide to woo physicians, it will have to face the same hurdles as the rEEG method, as well as possible stigma and hostility from the medical establishment resulting from its initial strategy.

1.8.2   Neurotherapy

Neurotherapy for the brain and nervous system is analogous to physical therapy for the body. The premise behind neurotherapy methods is that the behavior of the brain and nervous system can be modified in beneficial ways by exposing the patient to suitable stimuli and activities.

These therapies do not rely on, or prescribe, medications, but also do not conflict with the use of medications. There is no need for a patient to stop his medication in order to take advantage of these techniques (nor should he, without consulting the prescribing physician).

1.8.2.1   Chiropractic Neurology

Chiropractic Neurology is an outgrowth of the chiropractic approach to treating musculoskeletal disorders, but oriented towards the brain and nervous system. (For accreditation information, see www.acnb.org. Information about the treatment process is available at www.carrickinstitute.org). This specialty focuses on treating nervous-system disorders such as pain, sensory disorders, learning disorders, Tourette's Disorder, Attention Deficit-Hyperactivity Disorder, migraines, and mood disorders such as depression.

Assessment of the patient's condition is made by performing a variety of non-invasive tests of sensory function, blood pressure, coordination, sense of balance,

---

[3]Whether this situation is a good thing or a bad thing can doubtless be debated, but is not the focus here.

and other functions. Treatment consists of numerous physical techniques (similar to physical therapy), sensory techniques (periodic exposure to selected visual, auditory, and other stimuli), and so forth.

1.8.2.2   Neurofeedback

Neurofeedback is another neurotherapeutic approach. It is very similar in philosophy, and in the problems it treats, to chiropractic neurology (see www.eegspectrum.com). Assessment of the patient's condition is made largely through the use of electroencephalogram (EEG) recordings.

During treatment, the practitioner observe's the patient's responses with a real-time EEG display. The treatment uses a computer monitor to present games that encourage certain responses in the patient's brain. What the patient sees and does is influenced by the EEG signals, and vice versa (which is why this is a feedback technique). As the patient works to achieve certain goals in the game, he is also training his brain and nervous system to change in beneficial ways.

1.8.3   Conclusion

How these treatment strategies will play out over time is unknown. Neither correlation methods nor neurotherapy methods have yet been subjected to the level of clinical studies necessary to confirm how well they work. Until this type of scrutiny has been applied, an individual is left with at most anecdotal reports of success, and descriptions of underlying theory, as guides to evaluation.

The good news is that new strategies are becoming available to the people who have found the old strategies inadequate. There are times when necessity compels one to experiment with methods that have not been proven, because the alternative is unacceptable. At least these new methods are no more dangerous than current FDA-approved ones, and they show that new ideas are still appearing on the horizon.

1.9   Advice for the Patient (and Impatient)

The purpose of this book is to provide useful information, not to make recommendations for treatment. The only recommendations made here, for those who are suffering from mental illness, are these:

- Investigate medication and therapy with an open mind. You may need either or both. Only you can decide, but you need to be honest with yourself about what your problems really are.

- Find a good doctor. A psychiatrist is generally a better choice than a general practitioner, and a psychiatrist who specializes in psychopharmacology is a better choice still. Therapy can be very useful, but is often insufficient by itself. Medication is often required.

- Find a good therapist. The likelihood of success in the treatment of mental illness is greater when you get help from both therapy and medication. Medication can reduce the suffering, but therapy is often necessary to make changes in your life and behavior to solve the problems that cause or contribute to your condition.

- Be honest with your doctor and therapist about what is troubling you. Don't play games or hide the truth (or why bother talking to him in the first place?).

- Don't let an understandable reluctance to try medication that affects the functioning of your brain get in the way of your mental health. A bias against medication will not help you.

- If you read of a medication that seems particularly appropriate for your situation, discuss it with your doctor.

- If medication has not improved your mental health dramatically within twelve months (and you haven't been sabotaging yourself), get a second opinion from another doctor, preferably one who knows more than the one you've been seeing. It may be worth driving or flying 1000 miles to see a "high-powered" specialist for two hours, if you return home with new avenues to try that your physician hadn't thought of.

- If you don't have confidence in your doctor or therapist, find another one.

Above all else, perservere, educate yourself, and read on.

Chapter 2

Depression

The Web site for NAMI, the National Alliance for Mental Illness, at www.nami.org, describes Major Depression as follows:

> The symptoms of depression include:
>
> - persistently sad or irritable mood
> - pronounced changes in sleep, appetite, and energy
> - difficulty thinking, concentrating, and remembering
> - physical slowing or agitation
> - lack of interest in or pleasure from activities that were once enjoyed
> - feelings of guilt, worthlessness, hopelessness, and emptiness
> - recurrent thoughts of death or suicide
> - persistent physical symptoms that do not respond to treatment, such as headaches, digestive disorders, and chronic pain
>
> When several of these symptoms of depressive disorder occur at the same time, last longer than two weeks, and interfere with ordinary functioning, professional treatment is needed.

(It is the author's opinion that excessive anger, which does not abate, should also be added to this list, especially in the case of depression in men.)

Major Depression is severe and typically episodic. It may last weeks or months before fading away, then return months or years later.

Dysthymia is a term for mild chronic depression, which does not abate.

Double Depression refers to Major Depression experienced on top of Dysthymia.

The term *depression* will be used generically for both Major Depression and Dysthymia throughout.

Current medications for the treatment of depression, generally referred to as *antidepressant medications*, or *antidepressants*, work by increasing the concentration, in the brain, of one or more of these neurotransmitters: serotonin, norepinephrine, and dopamine.

2.1   Causes of Depression

Some symptoms of depression, such as melancholia (sadness), are common responses to unhappy experiences, such as the breakup of a close relationship, or death of a loved one. It is the persistence of the symptoms that characterizes the condition of Major Major Depressive Disorder as distinct from the sadder emotional fluctuations of a normal life.

Depression (meaning the disorder) may be triggered by external events (such as an emotional trauma), or simply appear for no obvious reason (in which case it is referred to as Endogenous Depression).

While the causes of depression at a neurological level remain unknown, there are reasons to believe that depression is related to abnormalities in brain chemistry, specifically the chemistry of neurotransmitter processes. One piece of evidence that supports this chemical imbalance hypothesis is the report of lower-than-normal levels of the neurotransmitter serotonin, found during autopsies in the brains of people who had been severely depressed at the time of death. Another piece of evidence is the empirical observation that medications that are known to influence neurotransmitter chemistry (especially by increasing neurotransmitter concentration) often alleviate depression.

It is not currently possible to measure neurotransmitter concentrations in the brains of living people, a limitation that makes analysis and treatment of depression more difficult than anyone likes. Nor (and largely as a result) is there any reliable way to connect specific neurotransmitter abnormalities in the brain to specific mood problems in an individual. Nevertheless, results trump theoretical discussions, and the fact is that most people who suffer from depression and seek medical treatment find that antidepressant medications alleviate their depression. In some cases, the alleviation is total and permanent, even after cessation of the medication. In some cases, the alleviation is partial, only happens while the medication is used, or both. In some individuals, unfortunately, existing medications do not alleviate depression, a painful fact that highlights the immaturity of the field, and the need for continuing research and development of better treatments for this life-destroying illness.

2.2   Treatments for Depression

Broadly speaking, the available treatments for depression fall into two general categories: Therapy and medical treatment. Some cases of depression can be resolved with therapy alone, while others can be resolved with medication alone. In general, though, success is more likely when therapy and medical treatment are combined.

The most effective technique for treating depression is that of electroconvulsive therapy, or ECT. This technique, which is described in Section 1.7.2, deserves careful consideration. Because of its drawbacks, ECT is not the method of choice for treating depression; however, it is effective, and worth considering if medication has failed.

The experimental treatments described in Section 1.8 may be of interest as well, although their effectiveness for depression has not yet been well established. However, the reader is advised to review these approaches in addition to the other techniques described below.

The following sections describe other medical treatments for depression that are in current use. The most common treatment strategy is that of antidepressant medications, which are discussed in more detail below.

2.2.1 Vagus-Nerve Stimulation (VNS)

The vagus nerve is one of 12 pairs of "cranial nerves," meaning nerves that originate in the brain. It is a very important nerve, one that is involved in motor functions (larynx, stomach, and heart) as well as sensory functions (ears, tongue), and so forth.

The technique of Vagus-Nerve Stimulation (VNS) was developed to treat epileptic seizures. An electric pulse generator (stimulator) is implanted in the chest, with a wire running up to the vagus nerve in the left side of the neck. The generator stimulates the vagus nerve with periodic pulses of programmed amplitude, duration, and frequency. This stimulation reduces the frequency of seizures.

While the effectiveness of VNS in treating seizures is well established, its usefulness in treating depression has been hotly contested. The Food and Drug Administration (FDA) approved VNS for the treatment of refractory (treatment-resistant) depression in 2005. However, the supporting evidence for this use is widely considered to be weak, and the decision produced much controversy.

Further research in the use of VNS to treat depression is necessary, but the lack of strong statistical indications of its effectiveness, combined with the expense and invasive nature of the device, makes this approach difficult to recommend at this time.

2.2.2 Transcranial Magnetic Stimulation (TMS)

Transcranial Magnetic Stimulation (TMS) is even more experimental, and less well-proven, than Vagus-Nerve Stimulation. Electromagnets placed outside the skull generate magnetic pulses of programmed amplitude, duration, and frequency. These time-varying magnetic pulses induce electric currents in targeted regions of the brain, stimulating them. There is some evidence to show that these pulses can alleviate depression in some people. The technique is an interesting one, and more appealing than ECT or VNS, as it does not cause seizures, require anesthesia, impair short-term memory, or require surgical implantation of any device.

This technique is far from proven at this time, and much progress needs to be made before it could be considered a reliable treatment for depression. However,

given its lack of invasiveness, there seems to be little drawback in trying the proce-
dure, if it is locally available.

2.2.3   Deep Brain Stimulation (DBS)

Deep Brain Stimulation (DBS) is a technique for treating neurological disorders
such as the symptoms (but not cause) of Parkinson's disease, and primary dystonia
(movement disorders). Surgery is used to implant electrodes in specfic areas in
the brain, connected to an implanted pacemaker device. The pacemaker generates
carefully-tailored electrical signals to the target areas of the brain, which serve to
alleviate the undesirable symptoms.

Preliminary research has indicated that DBS also alleviates depression in some
test subjects. Statistics are not available at this time to indicate how effective the
device is for treating depression, but the early results are promising. More research
is needed to determine how useful this approach will be to the general population.

Given the lack of information about its effectiveness, and considering its requirement for brain surgery, this technique cannot be recommended at this time.

2.2.4   Antidepressant Medication

Antidepressant medications come in a variety of categories, though all operate by
similar mechanisms (i.e., they modify neurotransmitter concentrations in the brain).
The reader would undoubtedly wish to know which medication, or category, is the
most effective in treating depression, but there is little that can be said in this regard.[1] For the most part, the different categories of medications are equally effective
in treating depression, with a success rate of approximately 33% (which means that
the average patient can expect to try two or three different medications before finding the most effective one for his or her case). The differences between the various
medications are not in their effectiveness, but in their side-effect profiles. Some categories (generally, the more modern medications) have fewer or less unpleasant side
effects than others, so that selection is often made as much on the basis of likely
side effects as any other reason.

The exception to the rule of uniform effectiveness is the category of Monoamine
Oxidase Inhibitors, described in Section 2.4. The MAO inhibitors are generally
regarded as somewhat more effective than the other categories, but are not often
prescribed, because of the drug interactions, food interactions, and dietary requirements that attend their use.

Psychiatrists tend to speak of MAO inhibitors much as they would speak of, say,
SSRIs (Selective Serotonin Reuptake Inhibitors), meaning as a category of medications with a very specific mechanism. However, this comparison is misleading. It is

---

[1]See Section 1.8.1.1 for an experimental technique that attempts to answer this question on an
individual basis.

more appropriate to speak of standard antidepressants as falling into two major categories, the reuptake inhibitors, and the MAO inhibitors. The reuptake inhibitors are distributed among many other classes, depending on which neurotransmitters they affect, their chemical structure, and so forth, but all exhibit the common mechanism of increasing the concentration of one or more neurotransmitters in the synaptic gap by blocking the re-absorption (reuptake) of neurotransmitters by the emitting neuron.

Similarly, the MAO inhibitors share the common mechanism of increasing the concentration of some neurotransmitters, by disabling the enzymes (Monoamine Oxidase) that destroy free-floating neurotransmitter molecules in the synaptic gap. However, the various MAO inhibitors fall into different sub-categories, with substantially different properties. The tendency to lump them all together into a single category is understandable but misguided. The differences are important.

It is a curious fact, doubtless driven at least in part by the phenomenal market success of Prozac, that the great majority of antidepressant medications act largely, or wholly, to boost the concentration of serotonin in the brain. Medications that increase the concentration of norepinephrine or dopamine are much less common, and medications that boost either of the latter without a concomitant increase in serotonin are few in number.

However, there is no particular reason to believe that serotonin should be singled out as the sole neurotransmitter whose tweaking is most likely to alleviate depression. The medication most likely to alleviate depression for a particular person is the one that affects the neurotransmitter(s) that are involved in that particular case of depression. (See Section 1.3 for a discussion of the connection between depressive symptoms and specific neurotransmitters.) While no widely-accepted test exists to identify the most appropriate medications for a particular person, the experimental technique of Section 1.8.1.1 may be worth investigating for this purpose.

While Section 1.3 may provide some rough indication as to which types of antidepressant medication are more likely to be effective for different depressive symptoms, the most reliable advice is to try a different category of medication if one or two in the first category don't work. There is likely to be little benefit to trying a third or fourth SSRI if the first or second don't work, and much greater likelihood that a medication that affects norepinephrine or dopamine will prove useful.

Warning! It is very important that anyone suffering from bipolar disorder (as in Chapter 3) *not* take any antidepressant that increases serotonin concentration (such as the SSRI, SNRI, TCA, and MAOI categories), without taking a mood-stabilizer medication at the same time. Taking one of these antidepressants without a mood stabilizer can trigger manic states. If you find that taking one of these antidepressants leads to excessive spending, grandiose behavior, hyperactivity and insomnia, consult your psychiatrist immediately. You may have bipolar disorder, and require an appropriate treatment for it.

Warning! As with all medications, an overdose of antidepressants can be dangerous. Overdose of medications that increase serotonin concentration can lead to a dangerous condition known as Serotonin Syndrome. This condition arises most frequently when people take two medications that both increase serotonin levels, not realizing that the effect on serotonin is cumulative.

2.3   Non-Prescription Antidepressants

While many non-prescription formulations might be considered candidates for the label "antidepressant" by people who have come to believe in them, only a few stand out as effective enough to be widely accepted. These medications do exist, however, and are worth considering as options for the treatment of depression. (Note that, as with all antidepressant medications, benefits may take from two to four weeks to become apparent.)

Motivations for trying non-prescription antidepressants include availability, cost, specific benefits (i.e., effectiveness and benign side-effect profile), and the belief, among some, that some of these medications are "natural" substances and therefore safer than prescription medications. While the author does not subscribe to the latter philosophy ("naturalness" does not guarantee absence of side effects), the other reasons are sufficient to justify consideration of these medications.

Most familiar non-prescription medications (such as allergy medicines) are widely accepted to produce the benefits for which they are sold. Such is not the case with the medications discussed in this section, none of which have FDA approval for any use. For this reason, these medications cannot legally be labeled as treating depression or other medical conditions, at least in the United States. However, while the reader should be aware of this fact, it is also true that a substance can be useful even though it lacks an FDA seal of approval.

The immediate practical benefit of most non-prescription antidepressants is their low cost. However, they also come with significant drawbacks, even if one assumes that they are generally effective. The most immediate drawback is the lack of reliable information about dosage. No firm guidelines are available as to amount per dose, and number of doses per day. Manufacturers typically supply suggestions, but these suggestions lack the weight of experience (and evidence) that inform the instructions for prescription medications. Thus the average consumer can easily take too little or too much of the medication, or take it at the wrong intervals. As a result, he may not experience the benefits the medication could provide if properly administered, or (even worse) experience only unpleasant effects.

The first rule for non-prescription antidepressants is *caveat emptor*: Let the buyer beware! Read as much as possible about the medication before taking it, to understand the pros, the cons, and the proper dosing.

2.3.1 Serotonin Precursors

A precursor is a chemical that is converted into another chemical of interest. More specifically, a serotonin precursor is any chemical that is converted, by one or more steps, into serotonin. Since prescriptions medications that increase serotonin concentration are often effective at treating depression, it makes sense that any mechanism that increases serotonin concentration is also a candidate for this purpose. Thus serotonin precursors, which are easily obtained without need for prescription, are often used to treat depression.

2.3.1.1 Mechanism

The immediate precursor to serotonin, which is converted directly into it, is 5-Hydroxytryptophan (5-HTP). Another chemical of interest, L-Tryptophan, is a precursor to 5-HTP, and thus also a serotonin precursor. Consumption of either 5-HTP or L-Tryptophan, therefore, can increase serotonin concentration in the body and brain.

The practical differences between 5-HTP and L-Tryptophan arise from the fact that the former passes more easily into the central nervous system, and its absorption is not affected by dietary factors. Thus the amount of serotonin produced is linked more closely to the amount of 5-HTP consumed, than to the amount of L-Tryptophan consumed, and the effects of 5-HTP manifest more rapidly.

2.3.1.2 Benefits

The serotonin precursors have relatively little in the way of side effects, as they are chemicals that naturally occur in both foods and the human body.

2.3.1.3 Principal Drawbacks

The serotonin precursors have short half-lives, which means their effects wear off quickly. Thus the effects of a single dose of L-Tryptophan, taken at bed time as a sleep aid, may wear off earlier than desired, and result in premature awakening.

The short half-lives have a more serious consequence for the treatment of depression. A dose of, say, 5-HTP, taken in the morning, will have completely disappeared from the body before bedtime, and its benefits may quickly follow. The result can be a roller-coaster ride of calmness alternating with depression and anxiety. In addition, the unpleasant symptoms can be even worse than normal, aggravated by the sudden decline in serotonin concentration.

Ideally, the serotonin precursors would be provided in a time-release formulation for steady release throughout a 24-hour cycle. In the absence of time-release formulations, one will typically need to take three doses per day, spaced uniformly.

Finally, people who have bipolar disorder should not take a serotonin precursor without also taking a mood stabilizer, since these medications can trigger manic episodes in people who have bipolar disorder (as can any medication that increases serotonin concentration).

2.3.1.4 Medications

Main Brand Name	Chemical Name	Chemical Type	Half Life	Wash-out Time	On-Label Uses	Off-Label Uses
5-HTP	5-Hydroxy-tryptophan		90 min-utes	8 hours	None (non-prescription medication)	Depression; Insomnia; overeating (as appetite suppres-sant)
Optimax	L-Trypto-phan		2 hours	10 hours	None (non-prescription medication)	Depression; Insomnia

2.3.1.5 Brand Names

Chemical Name	Brand Names (Principal in Bold)
5-Hydroxy-trypto-phan	**5-HTP**
L-Trypto-phan	**Optimax**

2.3.2 St. John's Wort

St. John's Wort is both a non-prescription medication, and the name of the plant from which it is derived. (The medication is often called *Hypericum*, from the Latin name for the plant. The term Hypericum will be used here as a shorthand for the active ingredients of St. John's Wort.) The preparation supplied to consumers (hereafter called SJW) consists of capsules or teas made from the flowering tops of the plant. Because of its preparation, SJW contains a complex mix of chemicals (including hyperforin, hypericin and biapigenin), and thus generates an equally complex set of chemical reactions in the body. Although commercial preparations often state the amount of hypericin per dose, hypericin is only one component of the mixture. The assumption is that other active ingredients will comprise fixed fractions of the dose, relative to hypericin, so that capsules with twice the amount of hypericin will also contain twice the amount of other active ingredients. This assumption is true only in the most approximate sense, and wide variations in proportions should be expected across manufacturers (indeed, some manufacturers deliberately change the proportions in an effort to improve effectiveness).

Clinical studies have shown that the effectiveness of SJW in treating depression is comparable to, or better than, Paroxetine, Fluoxetine, Sertraline, and Imipramine. At the same time, side effects from SJW are typically less troublesome than those of most prescription antidepressants.

2.3.2.1 Mechanism

The mechanism of SJW is not known (certainly less well known than for prescription medications), in part because standard preparations contain multiple active ingredients that work in different ways. Evidence exists that SJW inhibits reuptake of multiple neurotransmitters, including serotonin, norepinephrine, dopamine, GABA, and glutamate. It also appears to stimulate the release of adenosine and acetylcholine, and block NMDA receptors.

These observations must be considered preliminary, incomplete, and subject to revision by future research. What is clear is that SJW has many more effects on brain chemistry than does any of the prescription antidepressants. It is likely that the wide variety of effects contributes to the medication's effectiveness. In this regard, SJW somewhat resembles the early MAO inhibitors, which also have the reputation of being more effective than most other antidepressants. (Unlike SJW, MAO inhibitors are also more dangerous than other antidepressants.)

The half-life of SJW is difficult to estimate, as the different active ingredients have different half lives. The value usually quoted is the half-life of hypericin, which ranges from 26 to 42 hours (most sources use the figure of 26 hours).

2.3.2.2 Benefits

SJW is an effective antidepressant, with remarkably little in the way of unpleasant side effects. The combination of effectiveness and benign side-effect profile is unique among antidepressants. SJW has also been used to treat anxiety and somatoform disorder.

2.3.2.3 Principal Drawbacks

One problem that is unique to SJW, compared to prescription medications, is that its preparation is not rigidly controlled. The result is that capsules from one manufacturer may contain significantly different concentrations of effective elements than anothers. The buyer is advised to seek advice on reputable brands, and stay with a brand that has been found to be effective (and for which the individual's appropriate dose has been determined).

While side effects are usually absent or mild, they do exist, and can include anxiety, dry mouth, dizziness, gastrointestinal symptoms, fatigue, drowsiness, headache, and sexual dysfunction.

The major drawbacks to SJW are its potentially serious interactions with other medications. The National Center for Complementary and Alternative Medicine provides the following list of affected drugs (see nccam.nih.gov/health/stjohnswort):

- Indinavir and possibly other drugs used to control HIV infection

- Irinotecan and possibly other drugs used to treat cancer

- Cyclosporine, which prevents the body from rejecting transplanted organs

- Digoxin, which strengthens heart muscle contractions

- Warfarin and related anticoagulants

- Birth control pills

- Antidepressants

Caution should be exercised when taking SJW with a prescription antidepressant. The cumulative effect may be beneficial for depression, or may produce too much serotonin and cause serotonin syndrome. If symptoms of serotonin syndrome start to appear, reduce one or more of the antidepressant medications.

People who have bipolar disorder should not take SJW without also taking a mood stabilizer, since SJW can trigger manic episodes in people who have bipolar disorder (as can any medication that increases serotonin concentration).

2.3.2.4 Medications

Main Brand Name	Chemical Name	Chemical Type	Half Life	Wash-out Time	On-Label Uses	Off-Label Uses
St. John's Wort	Hypericum		26 hours	6 days	None (non-prescription medication)	Depression; anxiety; Somatoform Disorder

2.3.2.5 Brand Names

Chemical Name	Brand Names (Principal in Bold)
Hypericum	**St. John's Wort**, Saint John's Wort

2.3.3 SAM-e

SAM-e is an abbreviation for S-Adenosylmethionine, a chemical that is derived from the amino acid L-Methionine, and which occurs naturally in the body. SAM-e is involved in a variety of metabolic processes, including the production of norepinephrine and serotonin.

Clinical studies have shown that non-prescription SAM-e supplements can treat depression successfully, with an effectiveness comparable to prescription antidepressants, and relatively little in the way of side effects.

2.3.3.1 Mechanism

It is known that SAM-e is required for the production of norepinephrine and serotonin, so it is logical to conclude that SAM-e supplementation leads to an increase in the concentration of these two neurotransmitters. If so, then it may produce antidepressant effects for roughly the same reason as prescription medications such as Venlafaxine, which cause a similar increase, although by a different mechanism. However, this is only speculation, and the mechanism by which SAM-e alleviates depression is not known.

2.3.3.2 Benefits

SAM-e has been shown to be effective in the treatment of depression, and to relieve the pain of osteoarthritis as effectively as non-steroidal anti-inflammatory drugs (NSAIDs) such as aspirin and ibuprofen. (The latter benefit is particularly significant, as prolonged use of NSAID medications often causes significant damage to the stomach lining, occasionally to a fatal degree.) Since the chemical occurs naturally in the body, it has little in the way of side effects, so long as it is not taken to excess.

2.3.3.3 Principal Drawbacks

Theoretically, taking substantial amounts of SAM-e could cause an undesirable buildup of homocysteine (a natural metabolic product), though no such cases have been reported. If this is a concern, folate and vitamin B supplements can be taken to help metabolize homocysteine.

People who have bipolar disorder should not take SAM-e without also taking a mood stabilizer, since SAM-e can trigger manic episodes in people who have bipolar disorder (as can any medication that increases serotonin concentration).

2.3.3.4   Medications

Main Brand Name	Chemical Name	Chemical Type	Half Life	Wash-out Time	On-Label Uses	Off-Label Uses
SAM-e	S-adenosyl-methionine		100 minutes	8 hours	None (non-prescription medication)	Depression; Osteoarthritis (for pain)

2.3.3.5   Brand Names

Chemical Name	Brand Names (Principal in Bold)
S-adenosyl-methionine	**SAM-e**

2.4   Monoamine Oxidase Inhibitors (MAOI)

The Monoamine Oxidase Inhibitors were the first antidepressant family discovered (in the 1950s). These medications were discovered in a quest for improved tuberculosis treatments. They failed in that role, but were found to alleviate depression markedly in many patients. Though quite effective, as antidepressants go, MAO inhibitors are seldom used at the present time. The main reason for their infrequent use is that they can react with some medications and foods to cause a hypertensive crisis, a dramatic rise in blood pressure that can cause severe headaches, permanent injury, or death.

Physicians are understandably reluctant to prescribe medications that can harm their patients, especially if alternatives exist. However, it is perhaps unfortunate that the MAO inhibitors are so seldom offered to patients, given that they are quite effective as antidepressants. While no other antidepressants outperform MAO inhibitors, there is anecdotal evidence to suggest that MAO inhibitors outperform all other antidepressants for difficult cases.

The greater safety of reuptake inhibitors makes them the obvious choice for initial treatment, but MAO inhibitors are worth considering if the first few reuptake inhibitors fail to help.

This category of medication is receiving renewed interest as a result of the recent introduction of the Emsam transdermal (skin) patch, which supplies the MAO inhibitor Selegiline through the skin. Selegiline is a very effective antidepressant, and the patch's delivery mechanism bypasses the digestive tract, thus avoiding the food-interaction problems that have plagued this category of medication. The Emsam patch has revitalized MAO inhibitor therapy, which is excellent news for those who suffer from depression. (The off-label use of Selegiline for the treatment of sexual dysfunction, as described in Chapter 5, may further boost the popularity of this medication.)

2.4.1 Mechanism

MAOIs inhibit (deactivate) one or both types of monoamine oxidase (MAO), the enzymes that metabolize (destroy) neurotransmitters in the synaptic gap after signal transmission. Inhibition of neurotransmitter metabolization increases the concentration of neurotransmitters serotonin, norepinephrine, and dopamine (see Section 1.3 for details).

There are two types of MAO: MAO-A and MAO-B. MAO-A preferentially metabolizes serotonin and norepinephrine, and dopamine to a lesser extent. It is found primarily in the placenta, gut, and liver. MAO-B is found primarily in the brain, liver, and platelets. It breaks down only dopamine and phenylethylamine. Both MAO-A and MAO-B metabolize the amino acid tyramine, but MAO-A does so more strongly.

MAO Inhibitors work by bonding to monoamine oxidase molecules and therefore inactivating them, since the molecular bonds previously available to the enzyme for use in metabolizing neurotransmitters are no longer available for that purpose.

MAO Inhibitors may be selective (specific) or nonselective (nonspecific), and reversible or irreversible ("Reversible MAO Inhibitor" is sometimes abbreviated as RIMA).

Selective means that the MAOI inhibits only (or mostly) one of the two MAO types (A or B). Selectivity strongly influences the metabolization of tyramine, in that MAOI s that are selective for MAO-B are less likely to present dietary difficulties than the unselective type.

Reversible means that the bond between the MAOI molecule and the MAO enzyme can be broken, thus re-activating the MAO molecule, while "irreversible" means that the bond is permanent and cannot be broken. In the case of irreversible MAOIs, the return of MAO concentration to normal is limited by the body's ability to produce MAO to replace the missing quantities, a process that can take 10–14 days. In the case of reversible MAOIs, the MAO concentration should return to normal over approximately the same time scale as the drug's elimination from the body (i.e., a few half lives). However, the recommended washout time is typically nearly as long for the reversible as the irreversible MAOIs. The practical effect of reversibility appears to be that reversible MAOIs affect brain chemistry less strongly (i.e., are milder) than the irreversible versions, and do not require dietary restrictions (possibly because MAO binds more strongly to tyramine than the MAOI molecules).

A particular medication may have any combination of selectivity and reversibility. Since a particular MAOI drug might in principle affect either MAO-A or MAO-B or both, and, for each version it does affect, inhibit it either reversibly or irreversibly, there are eight possible categories of MAO inhibitors, as illustrated in the table below.

Effect on MAO-A	Effect on MAO-B	Abbreviation
Reversible	No effect	MAO-RA
No effect	Reversible	MAO-RB
Reversible	Reversible	MAO-RA,RB
Irreversible	No effect	MAO-IA
No effect	Irreversible	MAO-IB
Irreversible	Irreversible	MAO-IA,IB
Reversible	Irreversible	MAO-RA,IB
Irreversible	Reversible	MAO-IA,RB

The variety of possible actions should dispel the notion that MAO inhibitors represent one monolithic category. The effects of the different categories are quite distinct.

As of this writing, three of the eight possible categories correspond to available medications. These will be discussed in more detail below.

2.4.2   Reversible MAO-A Inhibitor (MAO-RA)

The selective inhibition of MAO-A produces an increase in the concentration of serotonin and norepinephrine in the brain.

Moclobemide is a reversible MAO inhibitor (RIMA), which is selective for MAO-A. At a 300 mg dose, the inhibition of MAO-A is approximately 80%, while the inhibition of MAO-B is approximately 20–30%. The MAO-A inhibition is both reversible and short-lasting (no more than 24 hours). Because the reaction with MAO-A is reversible, while the reaction between tyramine and MAO-A is not, the competition between Moclobemide and tyramine for MAO-A favors tyramine sufficiently that tyramine is metabolized by MAO-A even in the presence of Moclobemide. Thus even though Moclobemide is selective for MAO-A, it does not typically present any difficulties with food interactions.

2.4.2.1   Benefits

Moclobemide has no dietary restrictions, and relatively modest drug interactions. It may work better when combined with a tricyclic antidepressant or lithium.

2.4.2.2   Principal Drawbacks

Moclobemide's drawbacks stem from the same selectivity and reversibility that provide its benign lack of food and drug interactions. Because it affects only one of the two MAO enzymes, and because its chemistry is reversible, its effects are relatively weak. It is the least effective of all the MAO inhibitors in the treatment of depression.

2.4.2.3 Medications

Main Brand Name	Chemical Name	Chemical Type	Half Life	Wash-out Time	On-Label Uses	Off-Label Uses
Manerix	Moclo-bemide		90 min-utes	1 day	Depression	

2.4.2.4 Brand Names

Chemical Name	Brand Names (Principal in Bold)
Moclo-bemide	**Manerix**, Aurorix, Moclaime, Moclamide, Moclamine, Moclobemid, Moclobemida, Moclobemidum, Modobemde

2.4.3 Irreversible MAO-B Inhibitor (MAO-IB)

The selective inhibition of MAO-B produces an increase in the concentration of dopamine in the brain. Since dopamine is a precursor to norepinephrine, the increase in dopamine concentration leads directly to an increase in norepinephrine concentration as well.

The first (and for a long time, only) medication in this category was Selegiline. Selegiline was discovered in the 1960s, and initially approved by the Food and Drug Administration (FDA) for the treatment of Parkinson's disease. In 2006, Selegiline was finally approved for the treatment of depression, at which it is quite effective.

Selegiline is also used on an off-label basis for the treatment of sexual dysfunction resulting from lack of libido. Other off-label uses for Selegiline include the treatment of Alzheimer's disease, and the negative symptoms of schizophrenia.

Selegiline's unusual effectiveness for a wide variety of disorders, combined with its relative obscurity, make it perhaps the most under-prescribed psychotropic medication known. The good news is that the introduction of the Emsam skin-patch formulation of Selegiline is beginning to address this unfortunate obscurity.

Rasagaline, the newest medication in this category, was approved in 2006 for the treatment of Parkinson's disease. Because it shares the same primary mechanism as Selegiline, Rasagiline is likely to be useful for many of the same disorders, especially for depression and sexual dysfunction. However, this medication has not been in use long enough to provide a good understanding of off-label uses for which it may be appropriate.

Rasagiline is known to inhibit MAO-B. It is believed to inhibit only MAO-B, not MAO-A; however, conclusive proof has not yet been obtained to demonstrate that no MAO-A inhibition occurs. Until such proof becomes available, foods that contain tyramine should be avoided.

The chemistry of Selegiline is complex. At the lower doses typical of treatment for Parkinson's disease (10 mg orally), it irreversibly metabolizes MAO-B, and is a weak reversible inhibitor of MAO-A. Thus at these doses, tyramine ingestion is not a problem, and dietary restrictions are not required. At higher doses (20 mg or more, orally) typical for antidepressant use, Selegiline becomes an irreversible inhibitor of both MAO-A and -B, and has the same problems with tyramine as most of the MAOIs. (Selegiline is also unusual in that it has developed something of a cult following, with claims made that it improves thinking, increases intelligence, extends lifespan, and protects the brain against damage from oxidative damage, free radicals, ionizing radiation, and the illegal drug MDMA, known as "Ecstasy".)

2.4.3.1   Benefits

These are among the very few prescription medications that have a pronounced dopaminergic action, i.e., which give a powerful boost to the brain's dopamine chemistry (much more so than, say, Bupropion). Thus they are particularly effective at treating anhedonia and lack of libido, as libido, and the ability to feel pleasure, are both driven largely by dopamine chemistry. Also, because they does not increase serotonin concentration significantly in most cases, they do not actively suppress sexual performance or libido.

Eating foods that contain tyramine can cause a dangerous hypertensive crisis (episode of high blood pressure) for someone taking a medication that inhibits MAO-A. The medications of this section have as their primary mechanism the selective inhibition of MAO-B, which in principle eliminates this danger. Unfortunately, the reality is not quite this clear-cut (see Section 2.4.3.2 below), but it is true that these medications greatly reduce problems with tyramine compared to the non-selective MAO inhibitors.

While Selegiline does cause some MAO-A inhibition at higher doses, the degree to which effect this translates into danger of high blood pressure varies with the individual, and may not be significant for many people at doses of therapeutic use in the treatment of depression (for example, up to 40 mg orally).

The transdermal (skin patch) version of Selegiline supplies the medication gradually, through the skin. The gradual dispensation provides for a more constant level of medication in the body than does the oral form. Also, because it bypasses the gut, this delivery mechanism reduces or eliminates food interactions and dietary restrictions associated with the oral form.

2.4.3.2 Principal Drawbacks

The principal drawback of these medications are dangerous interactions with some other medications (something that is true for all irreversible MAO inhibitors). The most common of the dangerous medications are over-the-counter cold medications (decongestants, and cough medicine containing Dextromethorphan, but not anti-histamines), and the pain medicine Meperidine (Demerol). The combination of an MAO-B inhibitor with any of these medications can produce dangerous reactions such as increases in blood pressure, convulsions, and psychotic episodes.

Given the uncertainty around the possibility of tyramine interactions, the patient is strongly advised to purchase an inexpensive blood-pressure gauge and measure blood pressure before and after eating foods that contain tyramine (starting with small quantities), in order to understand his or her individual sensitivity. It is much better to know, than to guess and risk a hypertensive crisis.

Since Selegiline can cause MAO-A inhibition, some people who take Selegiline orally may experience an increase in blood pressure after eating foods that contain tyramine, especially at the higher doses. Monitoring of blood pressure in conjunction with eating these foods is recommended. The likelihood and severity of food interactions can be reduced further by taking an orally-dissolving formulation (Zelapar), or by using the transdermal (skin-patch) formulation (Emsam), both of which bypass the digestive tract.

2.4.3.3 Medications

Main Brand Name	Chemical Name	Chemical Type	Half Life	Wash-out Time	On-Label Uses	Off-Label Uses
Azilect	Rasagiline		3 hours	14 days	Parkinson's Disease	Depression; Sexual Dysfunction
Eldepryl	Selegiline (oral)		10 hours	14 days	Depression; Parkinson's Disease (Adjunctive)	Sexual Dysfunction; Alzheimer's Disease; Schizophrenia (negative symptoms)
Emsam	Selegiline (patch)		1 day	14 days	Depression	Sexual Dysfunction

2.4.3.4   Brand Names

Chemical Name	Brand Names (Principal in Bold)
Rasagiline	**Azilect**
Selegiline (oral)	**Eldepryl**, Apo-Selegiline, Atapryl, Carbex, Cyprenil, Deprenyl, Eldeprine, Gen-Selegiline, Jumex, Jumexal, Lesotal, L-Deprenalin, Movergan, Novo-Selegiline, Nu-Selegiline, Sd Deprenyl, Selegeline Hcl, Selegilina, Selegiline-5, Selegilinum, Selpak, Zelapar
Selegiline (patch)	**Emsam**

2.4.4   Irreversible MAO-A and MAO-B Inhibitor (MAO-IA,IB)

The non-selective inhibition of both MAO-A and MAO-B produces an increase in the concentration of serotonin, norepinephrine, and dopamine in the brain. The broad-spectrum boost in neurotransmitter chemistry provides a powerful antidepressant effect. It also provides for some of the negative side effects—this category of medications, like others that boost serotonin levels, tend to impair or suppress libido and sexual function.

Tranylcypromine is most often described as an irreversible inhibitor of both MAO-A and MAO-B, although there are a few references which contradict this assertion and claim that it is reversible. In any event, the washout times cited are more like those of irreversible MAO inhibitors, so it will be considered irreversible here.

2.4.4.1   Benefits

This category of MAO inhibitors represents the very first antidepressants discovered. They are often described as the most effective antidepressants known, and, for some, are the only ones that work.

2.4.4.2   Principal Drawbacks

These medicines are the antidepressants of last resort, rather than first, because they interact dangerously, even fatally, with foods that contain the amino acid tyramine (most cheeses, preserved meats, red wine, etc.) and numerous medications. Ingesting any of these foods or medications while taking this category of MAO inhibitor can cause a dramatic, painful, and even fatal skyrocketing of blood pressure (a hypertensive crisis). They also, as noted above, tend to reduce libido and sexual function.

While it makes a great deal of sense to first try antidepressants that are inherently safer than these, one should nevertheless not be frightened of this category if the safer medications prove inadequate. It is not difficult to avoid the troublesome foods and other medications, and their avoidance is a small price to pay for feeling good again. (However, one might want to start with the safer varieties of MAO inhibitors before trying this particular category.)

The burden of judging whether a particular food is safe can be reduced by purchasing a blood-pressure gauge, and checking blood pressure after meals that may contain some amount of tyramine. A blood-pressure gauge is also a good way to determine if a headache or other symptom indicates a hypertensive crisis, or is benign. Everyone who takes one of the medications in this category should own, and frequently use, one of these devices.

2.4.4.3 Medications

Main Brand Name	Chemical Name	Chemical Type	Half Life	Wash-out Time	On-Label Uses	Off-Label Uses
Marplan	Isocar-boxazid				Depression	
Nardil	Phenelzine		12 hours	10 days	Depression (especially Atypical, Non-endogenous, Neurotic), with anxiety, phobia, or hypochondria; Depression (Endogenous, less evidence of usefulness)	
Parnate	Tranyl-cypromine		2 hours	7 days	Depression (Major Depressive Episode without Melancholia)	

2.4.4.4   Brand Names

Chemical Name	Brand Names (Principal in Bold)
Isocar-boxazid	**Marplan**, BMIH, Benazide, Enerzer, Isocarbonazid, Isocarbossazide, Iso-carboxazida, Isocarboxazide, Isocarboxazidum, Isocarboxyzid, Maraplan, Marplon
Phenelzine	**Nardil**, Beta-phenylethylhydrazine, Fenelzin, Fenelzina, Fenelzyna, Fenelzyne, Kalgan, Monofen, Nardelzin, Phenalzine, Phenelezine, Phenelz-inum, Phenethylhydrazine, Phenylethyl hydrazine-HCl, Phenylethylhy-drazine, Stinerval
Tranyl-cypromine	**Parnate**, Dl-Tranylcypromine, Parmodalin, Sicoton, Transamin, Transamine, Transapin, Tylciprine

2.5   Reuptake Inhibitors

The second major category of antidepressant medications is the category of reuptake inhibitors. These medications were developed largely in reaction to the hypertensive dangers inherent in the MAO inhibitors. Reuptake inhibitors (of which the brand-name Prozac is undoubtedly the most famous) have been a tremendous success, bringing relief from depression to millions of people. The "Prozac revolution" put antidepressants on the map in the public mind, and forever changed the practice of psychiatry. That the revolution has had drawbacks (and that the medications have drawbacks) is indisputable, but also indisputable is the fact that those who suffer from depression have vastly more help available than was previously the case.

2.5.1   Mechanism

Reuptake inhibitors increase neurotransmitter concentrations by inhibiting the re-uptake of neurotransmitters emitted into the synaptic gap. Since less of the emitted neurotransmitter is absorbed by the emitting neurons, the concentration of the neu-rotransmitter in the synaptic gap increases (see Section 1.3 for details).

There is a wide variety of reuptake inhibitors to choose from. Some are catego-rized by molecular structure, and some by function. All of them inhibit reuptake for some combination of serotonin, norepinephrine, and dopamine. The medications vary widely in terms of their selectivity. Some inhibit reuptake of a single neuro-transmitter, while others inhibit the reuptake of two. As of this writing, none of the reuptake inhibitors strongly inhibit reuptake of all three of these neurotransmitters.

2.5.2   Tricyclic/Tetracyclic Antidepressants (TCA)

This category is named after the chemical structure of the medications, not for their mechanism. The medications are sometimes referred to as "second generation" antidepressants, although their discovery was contemporaneous with MAOIs. They are also known as *non-selective cyclic antidepressants*.

2.5.2.1 Mechanism

Most tricyclics suppress reuptake of serotonin and norepinephrine from the synaptic gap by the neuron that emitted them, thus increasing their concentration. They are not called SNRIs because the latter name is applied to newer medications, whose chemical structures are unrelated to the tricyclics.

Amoxapine not only suppresses reuptake of serotonin and norepinephrine, but blocks the response of dopamine receptors to dopamine (i.e., is a dopamine antagonist). (Note that dopamine antagonists are typically used for the treatment of psychosis.)

Amineptine, another tricyclic, is discussed in Section 2.5.10.

The site home.avvanta.com/~charlatn/depression/tricyclic.faq.html has this to say about the major classes of tricyclics:

> There are two broad chemical classes of tricyclics. The tertiary amines (amitriptyline, imipramine, trimipramine and doxepin), which have proportionally more effect in boosting serotonin than norepinephrine, produce more sedation, anticholinergic effects and orthostatic hypotension. Amitriptyline and doxepin are especially sedating. Secondary amines (nortriptyline, desipramine, and protriptyline) tend more toward enhancement of norepinephrine levels and hence toward irritability, overstimulation and disturbance of sleep. The tertiary amines, thus, are more useful where depression is accompanied by sleep disturbance, agitation and restlessness; whereas the secondary amines may be preferable where the depressed patient is fatigued, withdrawn, apathetic and inert. The psychiatrist's initial evaluation, therefore, must go into extensive detail about the pattern of depressive symptoms you have experienced, to tailor the agent to the condition. An impression about which side effects you would best tolerate (or even benefit from) will enter into the physician's choice of tricyclic as well. Overall, desipramine and nortriptyline are perhaps the most benign in terms of patient tolerance, and are often the initial tricyclic of choice.

2.5.2.2 Benefits

The tricyclics are effective antidepressants. The sedating tendency that many of them have can be useful when depression is accompanied by insomnia. Also, some of the tricyclics do not have the dramatic negative impact on sexual function for which the SSRIs (and other medications that increase serotonin concentration) are notorious, and can even be used to help resolve the problem. (See Section 5.3.4 for details.)

Protriptyline has an energizing effect, and may be particularly useful for those who suffer from fatigue and lack of energy.

2.5.2.3 Principal Drawbacks

The side effects of the tricyclics are substantially more unpleasant than those of the later-generation antidepressants, such as the SSRI drugs. As a result, they are now seldom prescribed for depression.

Typical problems are anticholinergic effects (dry mouth, urinary hesitation or retention, blurry vision, memory problems, or confusion), sedation (due to antihistamine properties), and weight gain. Other side effects that can occur include CNS toxicity, orthostatic hypotension, cardiovascular toxicity, and delirium. Like all medications that increase serotonin concentration, they may suppress libido and sexual performance, sometimes dramatically. (See Section 5.2 for ways to resolve these problems.)

Amoxapine exhibits some neuroleptic (antipsychotic) activity. As is often the case for neuroleptic medications, Amoxapine may, rarely, lead to Tardive Dyskinesia or Neuroleptic Malignant Syndrome. For these reasons, Amoxapine would not be a drug of first choice, and the physician and patient should be careful to note early symptoms of these two medical conditions and be prepared to stop administration of the medication immediately, should symptoms appear.

Warning! Maprotiline has the second-highest risk level (of four) for causing QT Prolongation and serious abnormalities of heart rhythm. Medications at this risk level have been associated with QT Prolongation, but not proven to cause it. The risk for QT Prolongation is not considered high, but medications with lower risk are preferred, especially for anyone who has Long QT Syndrome. If you cannot substitute a medication with lower risk, be alert for heart palpitations. If you experience palpitations, report them to your doctor immediately.

Note. Amitriptyline, Amoxapine, Clomipramine, Desipramine, Doxepin, Imipramine, Nortriptyline, Protriptyline, and Trimipramine have the lowest risk level (of four) for causing QT Prolongation and serious abnormalities of heart rhythm. Medications at this risk level are unlikely to cause problems when used at recommended dosage, but should be avoided by anyone who has Long QT Syndrome. However, be alert and report any heart palpitations to your doctor immediately.

2.5.2.4 Medications

All of these medications, except for Maprotiline are tricyclics, although Maprotiline is usually grouped with the tricyclics because of its similarity to them. Technically, Maprotiline is a *tetracyclic* (which still allows the use of the abbreviation TCA). Collectively, these medications may all be referred to as *hetero-cyclics*, but the term tricyclic is almost always used.

Main Brand Name	Chemical Name	Chemical Type	Half Life	Wash-out Time	On-Label Uses	Off-Label Uses
Anafranil	Clomip-ramine	Tricyclic	3 days	14 days	Obsessive-Compulsive Disorder	Depression
Asendin	Amoxapine	Tricyclic	24 hours	5 days	Depression; Psychotic Depression; anxiety	
Elavil	Amitrip-tyline	Tricyclic	20 hours	4 days	Depression	
Ludiomil	Maprotiline	Tetracyclic	2 days	10 days	Depression; Bipolar Disorder (Depressive phase); Psychotic Depression	
Norpramin	Desip-ramine	Tricyclic	1 day	5 days	Depression	
Pamelor	Nortrip-tyline	Tricyclic	20 hours	4 days	Depression	
Prothiaden	Dothiepin	Tricyclic	1 day	5 days	Depression; anxiety	Pain (from cancer); Fibromyalgia
Sinequan	Doxepin	Tricyclic	1 day	5 days	Depression; Psychotic Depression; anxiety	
Surmontil	Trimip-ramine	Tricyclic	1 day	5 days	Depression	
Tofranil	Imipramine	Tricyclic	19 hours	4 days	Depression	
Vivactil	Protrip-tyline	Tricyclic	16 days	80 days	Depression	

2.5.2.5   Brand Names

Chemical Name	Brand Names (Principal in Bold)
Amitrip-tyline	**Elavil**, Adepress, Adepril, Amitid, Amitril, Amitrip, Amitriproli-dine, Amitriptylin, Amitryptiline, Amitryptyline, Amytriptiline, Apo-Amitriptyline, Damilan, Damilen, Damitriptyline, Domical, Elanil, Emitrip, Endep, Enovil, Etravil, Flavyl, Hexathane, Horizon, Lantron, Laroxil, Laroxyl, Lentizol, Levate, Miketorin, Novotriptyn, Pinsanu, Proheptadiene, Quietal, Redomex, Saroten, Sarotex, Seroten, Sylvemid, Tridep, Tryptal, Triptanol, Triptilin, Triptisol, Triptizol, Tryptanol, Tryptizol, Uxen, Vana-trip
Amoxapine	**Asendin**, Amoxepine, Ascendin, Asendis, Defanyl, Demolox, Moxadil
Clomip-ramine	**Anafranil**, Chlorimipramine, Clofranil, Clomifril, Clomipramina, Clomipraminum, Clopress, Gromin, Hydiphen, Monochlorimipramine, Placil, 3-Chloroimipramine
Desip-ramine	**Norpramin**, DMI, Demethylimipramine, Desimipramine, Desimpramine, Desipramin, Desmethylimipramine, Dezipramine, Dimethylimipramine, Methylaminopropyliminodibenzyl, Metylyl, Monodemethylimipramine, Norimipramine, Norpramine, Nortimil, Pertrofane, Pentofran, Pertofran, Pertofrane, Pertofrin, Sertofran, Sertofren
Dothiepin	**Prothiaden**, Dosulepin, Dosulepine, Dothapax, Dothep, Prepadine, Thaden
Doxepin	**Sinequan**, Adapin, Aponal, Curatin, Desidox, Doneurin, Doxal, Doxedyn, Doxepina, Doxepine, Doxepinum, Novo-Doxepin, Poldoxin, Quitaxon, Tri-adapin, Zonalon
Imip-ramine	**Tofranil**, Antideprin, Apo-Imipramine, Berkomine, Censtim, Censtin, DPID, Declomipramine, Dimipressin, Dyna-Zina, Dynaprin, Estraldine, Ethipramine, Eupramin, IM, Imavate, Imidobenzyle, Imipramina, Imiprin, Imizin, Imizine, Imizinum, Impramine, Impril, Intalpram, Iramil, Irmin, Ja-nimine, Melipramin, Melipramine, Mipralin, Nelipramin, Norfranil, Novo-pramine, Pramine, Prazepine, Presamine, Promiben, Pryleugan, Psy-choforin, Sedacoroxen, Sk-Pramine, Surmontil, Surplix, Timolet, Tipramine, Tofranil-PM, Tofraniln A, Trimipramine Maleate, Venefon
Mapro-tiline	**Ludiomil**, Aneural, Deprilept, Maprotilina, Maludil, Maprotilinum, Maprotylina, Maprotylina, Melodil, Psymion, Retinyl
Nortrip-tyline	**Pamelor**, Acetexa, Allegron, Altilev, Ateben, Avantyl, Aventyl, Demethyl-Amitryptyline, Demethylamitriptylene, Demethylamitriptyline, Demethy-lamitryptyline, Desitriptilina, Desmethylamitriptyline, Lumbeck, No-ramitriptyline, Noritren, Nortrilen, Nortryptiline, Norzepine, Psychostyl, Sensaval, Sensival Ventyl, Sesaval, Vividyl
Protrip-tyline	**Vivactil**, Amimetilina, Anafranil, Apo-Amitriptyline, Apo-Imipramine, Apo-Trimip, Asendin, Aventyl, Impril, Levate, Norpramin, Novo-Doxepin, Novo-Tripramine, Novopramine, Novotriptyn, Pertofrane, Protryptyline, Rhotrimine, Surmontil, Tofranil, Triadapin 5, Triptil
Trimip-ramine	**Surmontil**, Apo-Trimip, Beta-Methylimipramine, Concordin, Concor-dine, Maximed, Novo-Tripramine, Rhotrimine, Sapilent, Trimeprimina, Trimeprimine, Trimipramina, Trimipraminum, Triptil

2.5.3 Selective Serotonin Reuptake Inhibitors (SSRI)

These SSRIs were developed in the hope that inhibiting reuptake of just a single neurotransmitter (serotonin) would avoid the unpleasant side effects of the MAOI and TCA medications. These medications are sometimes called the "third generation" family of antidepressants, although the first NDRI (Bupropion) was developed at about the same time.

2.5.3.1 Mechanism

SSRIs suppress reuptake of serotonin from the synaptic gap by the neuron that emitted them, thus increasing serotonin concentration.

Symbyax is a combination of the antidepressant Fluoxetine, and the atypical antipsychotic Olanzapine. This combination is sometimes more effective at treating symptoms of depression than Fluoxetine alone.

2.5.3.2 Benefits

The SSRIs are effective antidepressants. While they are no more effective at treating depression than the tricyclics they have largely replaced, their side effects are generally much less unpleasant. Similarly, the SSRIs do not have the problems of food and drug interactions common with the MAOIs. As a result, the SSRIs are used much more often than the tricyclics and MAOIs.

2.5.3.3 Principal Drawbacks

SSRIs may cause emotional "flatness," or flattened affect, that can be unpleasant. They usually suppress libido and sexual performance, sometimes dramatically. (See Section 5.2 for ways to resolve these problems.)

Withdrawal effects often arise when the medication is stopped. The withdrawal effects can be unpleasant, especially the peculiar "brain shock" feelings typical of SSRI withdrawal. Paroxetine is often cited as the worst offender in this regard. Withdrawal effects should be minimized by tapering slowly off the medication.

The side effects of Symbyax include those of both the antidepressant Fluoxetine (Section 2.5.3), and the atypical antipsychotic Olanzapine (Sections 4.3 and 4.5). The side effects are serious enough that use of Symbyax requires significant justification (i.e., other, safer medications have proven ineffective).

Warning! Venlafaxine has the second-highest risk level (of four) for causing QT Prolongation and serious abnormalities of heart rhythm. Medications at this risk level have been associated with QT Prolongation, but not proven to cause it. The risk for QT Prolongation is not considered high, but medications with lower risk are preferred, especially for anyone who has Long QT Syndrome. If you cannot substitute a medication with lower risk, be alert for heart palpitations. If you experience palpitations, report them to your doctor immediately.

Note. Citalopram, Fluoxetine, Paroxetine, and Sertraline have the lowest risk level (of four) for causing QT Prolongation and serious abnormalities of heart rhythm. Medications at this risk level are unlikely to cause problems when used at recommended dosage, but should be avoided by anyone who has Long QT Syndrome. However, be alert and report any heart palpitations to your doctor immediately.

2.5.3.4 Medications

Main Brand Name	Chemical Name	Chemical Type	Half Life	Washout Time	On-Label Uses	Off-Label Uses
Celexa	Citalopram	Bicyclic Phthalane derivative	35 hours	1 week	Depression	
Lexapro	Escitalopram	Citalopram derivative	30 hours	1 week	Depression; Generalized Anxiety Disorder	
Luvox	Fluvoxamine	Monocyclic	16 hours	3 days	Obsessive-Compulsive Disorder	Depression
Paxil	Paroxetine	Phenylpiperidine	21 hours	5 days	Depression; Obsessive-Compulsive Disorder; Panic Disorder (with or without agoraphobia); Social Anxiety Disorder; Generalized Anxiety Disorder; Post-Traumatic Stress Disorder	
Prozac	Fluoxetine	Bicyclic	1 week	5 weeks	Depression; Obsessive-Compulsive Disorder; Bulimia	
Symbyax	Fluoxetine + Olanzapine		1 week	5 weeks	Bipolar Disorder (Depressive phase)	Depression
Zoloft	Sertraline	Tetrahydronaphthylmethylamine	26 hours	1 week	Depression; Obsessive-Compulsive Disorder; Panic Disorder (with or without agoraphobia); Social Anxiety Disorder; Post-Traumatic Stress Disorder	

2.5.3.5   Brand Names

Chemical Name	Brand Names (Principal in Bold)
Citalo-pram	**Celexa**, Celexa, Cipram, Cipramil, Citalopramum, Nitalapram, Seropram
Escitalo-pram	**Lexapro**, Cipralex, Escitalopram Oxalate
Fluoxetine	**Prozac**, Adofen, Affectine, Animex-On, Ansilan, Deprex, Deproxin, Erocap, Eufor, Fluctin, Fluctine, Fludac, Flufran, Flunil, Fluoxeren, Fluoxac, Fluoxeren, Fluoxetina, Fluoxetina, Fluoxil, Fluoxetinum, Flutin, Flutine, Fluval, Fluxil, Fontex, Foxetin, Lorien, Lovan, Margrilan, Modipran, Neupax, Nopres, Oxedep, Portal, Pragmaten, Prizma, Prodep, Prozac Weekly, Pulvules, Reneuron, Rowexetina, Sanzur, Sarafem, Zactin, Zepax.
Fluoxetine + Olanza-pine	**Symbyax**
Fluvox-amine	**Luvox**, Avoxin, Depromel, Dumirox, Dumyrox, Faverin, Fevalat, Favoxil, Fevarin, Floxyfral, Fluvoxamina, Fluvoxamine maleate, Fluvoxaminum, Luvoxe, Maveral, Servox
Paroxetine	**Paxil**, Aropax, Deroxat, Lumin, Paroxetina, Paroxetinum, Paxil Cr, Pexeva, Pondera, Seroxat
Sertraline	**Zoloft**, Apo-Sertraline, Atruline, Lustral, Sertralina, Sertralinum, Sultamicillin Tosylate

2.5.4   Serotonin Antagonist/Reuptake Inhibitors (SARI)

2.5.4.1   Mechanism

SARIs suppress reuptake of serotonin from the synaptic gap by the neuron that emitted them, and also promote conversion of the serotonin precursor 5-HTP to serotonin (see Section 2.3.1). The result is to increase serotonin concentration. At the same time, they block the serotonin 5HT-2A receptor specifically, which reduces their negative impact on sexual function.

2.5.4.2   Benefits

These medications are effective antidepressants, and have the virtue of not suppressing libido and sexual function. They may even be used to alleviate sexual dysfunction caused by other antidepressants (see Section 5.3.4).

2.5.4.3   Principal Drawbacks

These medications may cause drowsiness and dizziness.

Nefazodone may cause life-threatening hepatic (liver) failure. This is a rare condition, with liver failure estimated to occur at a rate of one case per 250,000 patient-years. The prescribing physician should monitor the patient's liver function carefully and terminate the medication if signs of stress or injury appear. Nefazodone has been banned in some countries because of this problem.

Trazodone may cause priapism in men, a sustained and dangerous erection that can last for a day or more. It constitutes a medical emergency, and must be treated quickly by medication or surgery, to avoid permanent damage to the penis.

2.5.4.4 Medications

Main Brand Name	Chemical Name	Chemical Type	Half Life	Wash-out Time	On-Label Uses	Off-Label Uses
Desyrel	Trazodone	Triazolo-pyridine	12 hours	3 days	Depression	
Serzone	Nefazodone	Monocyclic	18 hours	4 days	Depression	

2.5.4.5 Brand Names

Chemical Name	Brand Names (Principal in Bold)
Nefazo-done	**Serzone**, Dutonin, Menfazona, Nefadar, Nefazodona, Nefazodonum, Nefirel, Reseril, Rulivan
Trazodone	**Desyrel**, Beneficat, Bimaran, Deprax, Desirel, Desyrel, Manegan, Molipaxin, Pragmarel, Pragmazone, Sideril, Taxagon, Thombran, Tombran, Trazalon, Trazodil, Trazodon, Trazodona, Trazodona, Trazodonum, Trazodonum, Trazolan, Trazonil, Trialodine, Trittico

2.5.5 Serotonin/Norepinephrine Reuptake Inhibitors (SNRI)

These medications were developed in the hope that inhibiting reuptake of two neurotransmitters (serotonin and norepinephrine) would be more effective than the SSRI medications, which inhibit reuptake of serotonin alone. Some studies show that the probability of medications in this category relieving depression is slightly, if not dramatically, higher than for the SSRIs.

2.5.5.1 Mechanism

SNRIs suppress reuptake of serotonin and norepinephrine from the synaptic gap by the neuron that emitted them, thus increasing their concentration.

In addition to strongly inhibiting reuptake of serotonin and norepinephrine, Duloxetine also weakly inhibits reuptake of dopamine.

2.5.5.2   Benefits

These medications are very similar to the SSRIs in terms of how they work, how they feel, and their safety. They are sometimes said to be more effective, because they increase the concentration of two neurotransmitters, instead of just one.

There have been anecdotal reports that Milnacipran is less likely to suppress libido or cause sexual dysfunction, the way SSRI medications and other SNRI medications do; however, it isn't clear why this should be the case.

2.5.5.3   Principal Drawbacks

The SNRI medications frequently suppress libido, and impair the ability to have orgasm (i.e., cause anorgasmia), even if libido and erectile function are present. (See Section 5.2 for details about why this problem occurs, and strategies to alleviate it.) The other most commonly reported side effects are nausea, diarrhea, or other gastrointestinal disorders, and insomnia.

Withdrawal effects often arise when the medication is stopped. The withdrawal effects can be unpleasant, especially the peculiar "brain shock" feelings typical of SNRI withdrawal. Venlafaxine is often cited as the worst offender in this regard. Withdrawal effects should be minimized by tapering slowly off the medication.

2.5.5.4   Medications

Main Brand Name	Chemical Name	Chemical Type	Half Life	Wash-out Time	On-Label Uses	Off-Label Uses
Cymbalta	Duloxetine		12 hours	3 days	Depression	Urinary Incontinence in Women
Dalcipran	Milnacipran	Tricyclic	8 hours	2 days	Depression	
Effexor	Venlafaxine	Bicyclic	16 hours	3 days	Depression; Generalized Anxiety Disorder; Social Anxiety Disorder	

2.5.5.5 Brand Names

Chemical Name	Brand Names (Principal in Bold)
Duloxetine	**Cymbalta**, Domperidone, Yentreve
Milnaci-pran	**Dalcipran**, Ixel
Venla-faxine	**Effexor**, Efexor, Effexor Xr, Elafax, Trevilor, Vandral, Venlafaxina

2.5.6 Norepinephrine Reuptake Inhibitors (NRI)

2.5.6.1 Mechanism

NRIs suppress reuptake of norepinephrine from the synaptic gap by the neuron that emitted them, thus increasing norepinephrine concentration.

2.5.6.2 Benefits

NRI medications are energizing, and improve the ability to concentrate. They have relatively little in the way of unpleasant side effects.

Stimulants (see Section 2.8) also increase norepinephrine concentration, boost energy, and improve concentration, but the mechanisms by which they do so are very different from the reuptake inhibitors in this category. Stimulants cause neurons to increase the rate at which they emit norepinephrine, while reuptake inhibitors reduce the rate at which norepinephrine is re-absorbed by the emitting neuron. Thus the reuptake inhibitors do not produce the negative effects of tolerance and addiction that are characteristic of stimulants. They are intrinsically more benign, better tolerated, and, because they are not controlled substances, easier to obtain.

2.5.6.3 Principal Drawbacks

Side effects are typically minor, and include decreased appetite, irritability, cough.

Warning! Atomoxetine has the third highest risk level (of four) for causing QT Prolongation and serious abnormalities of heart rhythm. Medications at this risk level should be avoided by anyone who has Long QT Syndrome, but should otherwise be safe. However, be alert and report any heart palpitations to your doctor immediately.

2.5.6.4   Medications

Main Brand Name	Chemical Name	Chemical Type	Half Life	Wash-out Time	On-Label Uses	Off-Label Uses
Edronax	Reboxetine	Tricyclic	12 hours	3 days	Depression	
Strattera	Atomoxe-tine		5 hours	1 day	Attention Deficit Hyperactivity Disorder	Depression

2.5.6.5   Brand Names

Chemical Name	Brand Names (Principal in Bold)
Atomoxe-tine	**Strattera**, Tomoxetina, Tomoxetine, Tomoxetine, Tomoxetinum
Reboxetine	**Edronax**, Norebox, Reboxetinemesylate, Vestra

2.5.7   Norepinephrine/Dopamine Reuptake Inhibitors (NDRI)

The only member in this category as of this writing, Bupropion (Wellbutrin), was developed at about the same time as the first SSRI (Fluoxetine, or Prozac). Unfortunately, early users of Bupropion were found to be more prone to seizures than the general population. Bupropion was reformulated into a sustained-release version that reduced the seizure incidence to roughly normal levels, but its history scared off physicians for many years. As a result, SSRIs, and especially Prozac, dominated the market for several years. After it became clear that Bupropion seldom decreases libido, and can even counteract the libido-suppression of SSRI medications when taken concurrently, its popularity surged. At this time, Bupropion is commonly prescribed.

2.5.7.1   Mechanism

NDRIs suppress reuptake of norepinephrine and dopamine from the synaptic gap by the neuron that emitted them, thus increasing their concentration.

2.5.7.2   Benefits

This medication is effective in treating depression. Unlike the SSRIs and most other antidepressant categories, it does not normally suppress libido. Bupropion is often prescribed along with SSRIs to alleviate the libido-suppression effects of SSRIs. This category has become increasingly popular as the libido issues have become better understood. (Bupropion is also prescribed as an aid in smoking cessation, under the name Zyban.)

2.5.7.3 Principal Drawbacks

Side effects include anxiety, jitteriness, insomnia, and increased possibility of seizures for seizure-prone populations (e.g., people with epilepsy).

2.5.7.4 Medications

Main Brand Name	Chemical Name	Chemical Type	Half Life	Wash-out Time	On-Label Uses	Off-Label Uses
Wellbutrin	Bupropion	Bicyclic	21 hours	8 days	Depression; Nicotine Addiction	Sexual Dysfunction (Anti-depressant-induced)

2.5.7.5 Brand Names

Chemical Name	Brand Names (Principal in Bold)
Bupropion	**Wellbutrin**, Wellbatrin, Zyban

2.5.8 Noradrenergic/Specific Serotonergic Antidepressants (NaSSA)

2.5.8.1 Mechanism

NaSSA medications increase the release of norepinephrine and serotonin, and block two specific serotonin receptors.

2.5.8.2 Benefits

These medications not only treat depression, but are particularly benign with respect to the kind of side effects that typically accompany medications that increase serotonin concentration. Blockage of the serotonin receptors reduces the negative impact on sexual function, and results in less nausea, nervousness, and diarrhea compared to SSRIs. This type of medication may even be used to alleviate sexual dysfunction caused by other antidepressants (see Section 5.3.4).

2.5.8.3   Principal Drawbacks

Side effects include drowsiness, increased appetite, weight gain, dizziness, dry mouth, and constipation.

A very small number in clinical trials for Mirtazapine (two out of 2796) developed agranulocytosis (drop in white-blood cell count, increasing vulnerability to infection), though it isn't clear that there was any connection with the medication. However, if symptoms of infection (sore throat, fever, mouth sores) develop while on this medication, they should be reported to a physician immediately.

2.5.8.4   Medications

Main Brand Name	Chemical Name	Chemical Type	Half Life	Wash-out Time	On-Label Uses	Off-Label Uses
Remeron	Mirtazapine	Tetracyclic	30 hours	1 week	Depression	

2.5.8.5   Brand Names

Chemical Name	Brand Names (Principal in Bold)
Mirtaza-pine	**Remeron**, Avanza, Axit, Mepirzepine, Mirtabene, Mirtaz, Mirtazapina, Mirtazapinum, Mirtazepine, Norset, Olsalazine, Remergil, Remergon, Remeron Soltab, Rexer, Zispin

2.5.9   Serotonin Reuptake Accelerators (SRA)

2.5.9.1   Mechanism

Medications in this category accelerate the reuptake of serotonin. It is counterintuitive that a reuptake *accelerator* would act as an antidepressant, given that serotonin reuptake inhibitors (SSRIs) are the most well-known antidepressants. One might expect an SRA to be a "depressant." Nevertheless, the sole entry in this category, Tianeptine (an atypical tricyclic antidepressant related to Amineptine) does alleviate depression.

Why Tianeptine relieves depression is not clear. Part of the reason may have to do with the fact that a decrease in serotonin concentration produces an increase in dopamine concentration, which can help some cases of depression.

2.5.9.2 Benefits

This medication is effective in treating depression. Because this type of medication reduces serotonin concentration, it should not cause sexual dysfunction, and may help to alleviate sexual problems. Other serotonergic side effects (nausea, nervousness, and diarrhea) should also be less common than with the SSRIs.

2.5.9.3 Principal Drawbacks

Side effects include nausea, constipation, abdominal pain, headache, dizziness, and changes in dreaming.

2.5.9.4 Medications

Main Brand Name	Chemical Name	Chemical Type	Half Life	Wash-out Time	On-Label Uses	Off-Label Uses
Stablon	Tianeptine	Tricyclic	3 hours	1 day	Depression	

2.5.9.5 Brand Names

Chemical Name	Brand Names (Principal in Bold)
Tianeptine	**Stablon**, Ardix

2.5.10 Dopamine Reuptake Inhibitors (DRI)

2.5.10.1 Mechanism

Amineptine is a dopamine reuptake inhibitor, and also promotes dopamine release at higher dosages. It stimulates the adrenergic system. Its antidepressant effects are similar to the other tricyclic antidepressants (TCAs), but it acts more rapidly, and is better tolerated (in terms of the usual side effects).

Amineptine can produce effects similar to psychomotor stimulants, such as amphetamines. It sometimes has the odd effect of causing spontaneous orgasms. It does not act on serotonin, and does not impair libido as SSRIs do.

2.5.10.2 Benefits

Amineptine has none of the serotonergic effects (e.g., loss of libido, sexual dysfunction) typical of SSRIs. In fact, it improves sexual dysfunction present in some patients. It is also reputed to improve quality of sleep.

2.5.10.3   Principal Drawbacks

Amineptine has a higher-than-normal risk for hepatotoxicity (liver damage), and,
largely for this reason, is not available in many countries. There have also been
claims that it is addictive, in the same sense that amphetamines are addictive,
because of its psychomotor stimulant effects, and these claims have undoubtedly
influenced the medication's availability (or lack thereof).

Other effects include gastralgia, abdominal pain, dryness of the mouth, anorexia,
nausea, vomiting, flatulence; insomnia, drowsiness, nightmares, asthenia; tachycar-
dia, extrasystole, precordialgia; dizziness, headaches, faintness, trembling, upsets;
respiratory discomfort, tightness of the throat; myalgia, and lumbago.

2.5.10.4   Medications

Main Brand Name	Chemical Name	Chemical Type	Half Life	Wash-out Time	On-Label Uses	Off-Label Uses
Survector	Amineptine	Tricyclic	8 hours	2 days	Depression	

2.5.10.5   Brand Names

Chemical Name	Brand Names (Principal in Bold)
Aminep-tine	**Survector**, Maneon, Directim

2.6   Medications for Bipolar Disorder

Some of the medications used to treat bipolar disorder have been found useful in
treating depression as well, usually as adjunctive medications (taken along with an
antidepressant). Lithium and Lamotrigine are perhaps the most commonly used for
this purpose. Chapter 3 describes these medications in more detail.

2.7   Dopamine Agonists (DA)

This section differs from most in this chapter in that none of the medications described have been approved by the Food and Drug Administration (FDA) as a
treatment for depression. The use of dopamine agonists to treat depression is still
experimental. However, sufficiently dramatic results have been achieved in some
cases to warrant a discussion of these medications in the context of treating depression. Based on the evidence available to date, and given that these medications are

not considered unusually dangerous, the author has concluded that they merit serious consideration as treatments for depression in situations where other approaches have been unsuccessful.

2.7.1 Mechanism

The neurotransmitter dopamine is heavily involved in the subjective experience of pleasure, and the capacity for libido (sexual desire). Some standard antidepressants achieve their results in part by increasing the concentration of dopamine, either by inhibiting its reuptake, or inhibiting its destruction by Monoamine Oxidase. Thus it is not surprising that a dopamine agonist, which can be thought of as supplying a replacement (agonist) for dopamine, would also act to increase the capacity for pleasure and sexual desire, in those whose capacity has been diminished by depression. In this context, dopamine agonists serve as a treatment for Anhedonia and sexual dysfunction (see Chapter 5).

The principle on-label uses of dopamine agonists are treatment for Parkinson's disease (usually in conjunction with l-dopa), and hyperprolactinemia. In the case of Parkinsons disease, dopamine agonists act to supplement the decreasing supply of dopamine in the brain. In the case of hyperprolactinemia, dopamine agonists act to suppress production of prolactin by the pituitary gland. This latter action can also result in shrinkage of pituitary gland tumors, when the illness is due to such a tumor.

Amantadine is known as an *indirect* dopamine agonist, because it does not act directly as a dopamine replacement. For this reason, it is also the weakest of the of the dopamine agonists. The mechanism by which Amantadine affects neurotransmitter chemistry is unknown; however, there is some evidence to suggest that it does one or both of the following: (1) Enhances dopamine concentration by increasing release, or decreasing reuptake, of dopamine; and (2) Stimulates the dopamine receptors directly, or makes the receptors more sensitive to dopamine. However, these suggested mechanisms are not regarded as reliably understood at this point.

2.7.2 Benefits

Anecdotal reports indicate an improved capacity for positive emotions, and improved libido, for individuals in whom these capacities are reduced by depression.

Perhaps because of its long half life (which minimizes fluctuations in blood levels), Cabergoline is least likely of all dopamine agonists to cause severe nausea, and is tolerated more easily than the others. One study showed that it had one third of the discontinuation rate (due to adverse side effects of nausea and headache) of Bromocriptine.

2.7.3   Principal Drawbacks

Dopamine agonists frequently cause nausea, headaches, and a variety of less common side effects. Nausea and headache are the two symptoms most likely to result in discontinuation of the medication.

Warning! Amantadine has the second-highest risk level (of four) for causing QT Prolongation and serious abnormalities of heart rhythm. Medications at this risk level have been associated with QT Prolongation, but not proven to cause it. The risk for QT Prolongation is not considered high, but medications with lower risk are preferred, especially for anyone who has Long QT Syndrome. If you cannot substitute a medication with lower risk, be alert for heart palpitations. If you experience palpitations, report them to your doctor immediately.

Warning! Bromocriptine, Pergolide, Pramipexole, and Ropinirole have been identified as causing people to fall asleep suddenly, without warning signs such as drowsiness, even as late as a year after initiating treatment. Anyone taking any of these medications should exercise care in driving and other circumstances where sudden sleep would be hazardous, until it has been established that this problem is unlikely to occur.

2.7.4 Medications

Main Brand Name	Chemical Name	Chemical Type	Half Life	Wash-out Time	On-Label Uses	Off-Label Uses
Dostinex	Cabergoline		3 days	15 days	Hyper-prolactinemia	Depression; Sexual Dysfunction
Mirapex	Prami-pexole		8 hours	2 days	Parkinson's Disease	Depression; Sexual Dysfunction
Parlodel	Bromo-criptine	Ergot derivative	1 day	5 days	Acromegaly; Hyper-prolactinemia; Parkinson's Disease	Depression; Sexual Dysfunction
Permax	Pergolide	Ergot derivative	24 hours	5 days	Parkinson's Disease (adjunctive)	Depression; Sexual Dysfunction
Requip	Ropinirole		6 hours	2 days	Parkinson's Disease	Depression; Sexual Dysfunction
Symmetrel	Amantadine		17 hours	4 days	Parkinson's Disease; Viral Infection (Influenza Type A)	Depression; Sexual Dysfunction
Trivastal	Piribedil		21 hours	5 days	Parkinson's Disease	Depression; Sexual Dysfunction

2.7.5   Brand Names

Chemical Name	Brand Names (Principal in Bold)
Amanta-dine	**Symmetrel**, Adamantamine, Adamantanamine, Adamantylamine, Amantidine, Aminoadamantane, Endantadine, Gen-Amantadine, Mantadine, Pk-Merz, Symadine
Bromo-criptine	**Parlodel**, Alti-Bromocriptine, Apo-Bromocriptine, Bromergocryptine, Bromocriptin, Bromocriptina, Bromocriptinum, Bromocryptine, Bromoergocriptine, Bromoergocryptine
Caber-goline	**Dostinex**, Cabaser, Cabergolina, Cabergolinum, Dostinex
Pergolide	**Permax**, Pergolida, Pergolide Mesylate, Pergolide Methanesulfonate, Pergolidum
Piribedil	**Trivastal**, Pronoran
Prami-pexole	**Mirapex**, Furfuryl Acetate, Pramipexol, Pramipexol, Pramipexolum, SUD919CL2Y
Ropinirole	**Requip**, Ropinirol, Ropinirolum

2.8   Stimulants

Stimulants represent another category of medication that has not been approved by the Food and Drug Administration (FDA) as a treatment for depression; however, the use of stimulants for this purpose is becoming increasingly common. Stimulants are used as an adjunctive therapy, in combination with more traditional antidepressants.

The major FDA-approved use of stimulants is for the treatment of Attention Deficit Hyperactivity Disorder (ADHD).

Why use stimulants to treat depression? Simply because, in a small subset of patients, adding stimulants to an antidepressant regimen has been found to alleviate depression when other approaches have failed. Thus while stimulants would not be a first-line (or monotherapy) treatment for depression, there are times when their use as an adjunctive therapy does help.

Stimulants are most likely to provide benefits for cases of depression where inability to feel pleasure (anhedonia) and lack of energy (anergia) are major problems. Whether they are the best choice for treating these conditions is an evaluation the physician must make in light of the patient's condition, and of alternative treatments available.

2.8.1   Mechanism

The standard CNS stimulants increase activity in the central nervous system. They are thought to block the reuptake of norepinephrine and dopamine, and to increase the total amounts of these neurotransmitters released from storage vesicles in the neurons. The result is to increase the concentration of norepinephrine and dopamine in the synaptic gap.

Medications that increase dopamine activity typically improve anhedonia and lack of libido, while medications that increase norepinephrine typically increase energy. Thus it is not surprising that stimulants can improve both mood and energy.

The mechanism by which stimulants alleviate ADHD is not known, but it appears that increasing norepinephrine concentration not only provides additional energy, but improves the ability to concentrate. Thus it makes sense that norepinephrine-reuptake inhibitors (NRIs) are also prescribed for ADHD (see Section 2.5.6).

However, given that safer medications exist that are non-addictive and produce stimulating effects (by increasing concentration of the relevant neurotransmitters), it makes sense to investigate the alternatives first. (Modafinil, which is not addicting, and which works by different mechanism than the standard CNS stimulants, is an exception. Modafinil's more benign behavior makes it the most appealing candidate, among the stimulants, for treating depression.)

An NRI medication, possibly in conjunction with a dopamine agonist (Section 2.7), provides one alternative to CNS stimulants. Another is the irreversible MAO-B inhibitor, Selegiline (Section 2.4.3), which may be taken in conjunction with a dopamine agonist, if necessary. If neither of these alternatives proves useful, stimulants would then be more attractive.

Lisdexamfetamine has no direct effects on the nervous system. However, it is a "pro-drug" of the stimulant dextroamphetamine, which means that it is converted to the latter in the body. As this conversion takes time, the overall effect is to provide a time-release mechanism for dextroamphetamine.

The mechanism by which Modafinil promotes wakefulness is not known, but is known to be different from that of amphetamines. Although Modafinil is known to increase dopamine concentration by inhibiting dopamine reuptake, the increase in dopamine concentration is not responsible for the improvement in wakefulness. (However, it would not be surprising if the dopaminergic effects contributed to alleviating depression, among those taking the medication for anti-depressant benefits.)

2.8.2 Benefits

Stimulants increase energy, improve the ability to focus (if not taken to excess), promote wakefulness, and often decrease appetite. The first two attributes are clearly beneficial to depressed people who lack energy and find it difficult to concentrate. The decrease in appetite and increase in wakefulness may be benefits or drawbacks, depending on circumstances.

The time-release effect provided by Lisdexamfetamine increases the duration of the medication's usefulness, compared to taking Dextroamphetamine directly. This formulation may also have less potential for addiction than Dextroamphetamine.

Modafinil's benefits consist largely of the absence of drawbacks associated with standard stimulants, such as Methylphenidate and the Amphetamines. In particular, Modafinil is not addictive, and is generally more benign in terms of its side effects.

Pemoline has a relatively low potential for addiction, and is classified as a Schedule-IV controlled substance.

2.8.3   Principal Drawbacks

Most stimulants (excepting Modafinil, for which the following drawbacks do not apply) have a high potential for addiction, and are therefore categorized by the Drug Enforcement Administration (DEA) as Schedule-II controlled substances. Medications in this category require a more tightly-regulated prescription process than do most medications.

Addiction in the narrow sense of chemical dependence, and vulnerability to withdrawal symptoms are significant issues, but not by themselves dangerous, in a therapeutic context. More dangerous is the potential for abuse by those who become addicted to stimulant-induced "highs," and seek greater effects by taking higher doses. Abuse of stimulants by deliberate overdosing can cause psychotic episodes, as well as other unfortunate effects (such as coma and death). Not everyone who takes stimulants experiences "highs," but those who do are at more risk than those who do not.

The benefit of stimulants can be short-lived. They act in part by inducing neurons to release neurotransmitters from storage vesicles at a greater-than-normal rate. The stimulated rate of emission can exceed the rate at which the neurons are capable of producing the neurotransmitters. If so, then the stimulant will stop working at the current dose. Increasing the dose at this point may boost the release and production rates, or, if the neurons are overtaxed, have no useful effect. At this point the person taking the stimulant may "crash," feeling suddenly fatigued, depressed, and ill, possibly to extreme degrees.

Abuse of Pemoline (as by deliberate overdosing) can cause psychotic episodes. More significantly, patients taking Pemoline have experienced acute hepatic (liver) failure at 4–17 times the average rate. Of the 15 reported cases between 1975 and 1998, 12 resulted in death or liver transplantation. The earliest onset of liver abnormalities occurred six months after initiation of Pemoline. Because of this increased risk for liver damage, Pemoline should not normally be considered for first-line drug therapy. If Pemoline is prescribed, the patient's liver function should be monitored periodically. (The reader should be aware that Pemoline has been withdrawn from the market in the United States, because of this issue.)

Warning! Amphetamines and Methylphenidate have the third highest risk level (of four) for causing QT Prolongation and serious abnormalities of heart rhythm. Medications at this risk level should be avoided by anyone who has Long QT Syndrome, but should otherwise be safe. However, be alert and report any heart palpitations to your doctor immediately.

2.8.4   Medications

Main Brand Name	Chemical Name	Chemical Type	Half Life	Wash-out Time	On-Label Uses	Off-Label Uses
Adderall	Amphetamine (mixture)	Amphetamine	12 hours	3 days	Attention Deficit Hyperactivity Disorder; Narcolepsy	Depression (Adjunctive)
Cylert	Pemoline		12 hours	3 days	Attention Deficit Hyperactivity Disorder	Depression (Adjunctive)
Dexedrine	Dextro-amphetamine	Amphetamine	12 hours	3 days	Attention Deficit Hyperactivity Disorder; Narcolepsy	Depression (Adjunctive)
Provigil	Modafinil		15 hours	3 days	Narcolepsy	Depression (Adjunctive)
Ritalin	Methyl-phenidate		3 hours	14 hours	Attention Deficit Hyperactivity Disorder; Narcolepsy	Depression (Adjunctive)
Vyvanse	Lisdexam-fetamine	Amphetamine	15 hours	3 days	Attention Deficit Hyperactivity Disorder	Depression (Adjunctive)

2.8.5   Brand Names

Chemical Name	Brand Names (Principal in Bold)
Amphet- amine (mixture)	**Adderall**
Dextro- amphet- amine	**Dexedrine**, Actedron, Adipan, Allodene, Amphetamine, Anorexide, Anorexine, Benzebar, Benzedrine, Benzolone, Deoxy-Norephedrine, DL-alpha-Methylphenethylamine, Desoxyn, Dexampex, Dextroamphetamine Sulfate, Dextrostat, Elastonon, Fenamin, Fenylo-izopropylaminyl, Ferndex, Finam, Isoamycin, Isoamyne, Isomyn, Mecodrin, Methampex, Methamphetamine HCL, Norephedrane, Novydrine, Oktedrin, Ortedrine, Paredrine, Percomon, Phenamine, Phenedrine, Phenylisopropylamine, Profamina, Propisamine, Psychedrine, Raphetamine, Rhinalator, Simpatedrin, Simpatina, Sympamin, Sympamine, Sympatedrine, Weckamine, [1-(3-Methoxyphenyl)-2-propyl]amine, Alpha-Methylbenzeneethaneamine, Beta-Aminopropylbenzene, Dl-1-Phenyl-2-aminopropane, Dl-Amphetamine, Dl-Benzedrine, M-Methoxy-a-methylphenethylamine, M-Methoxyamphetamine, Racemic-Desoxynorephedrine,(+/-)-Benzedrine, (+/-)-Desoxynorephedrine, (+/-)-beta-Phenylisopropylamine, 1-Methyl-2-phenylethylamine, 1-Phenyl-2-aminopropane, 3-Methoxy-a-methylbenzeneethanamine, 3-Methoxyamphetamine, 3-Methoxyphenylisopropylamine
Lisdexam- fetamine	**Vyvanse**
Methyl- phenidate	**Ritalin**, 4311/B Ciba, Calocain, Centedein, Centedrin, Centedrine, Centredin, Concerta, Focalin, Focalin XR, Methylphen, Meridil, Metadate, Metadate CD, Metadate ER, Methyl phenidyl acetate, Methylin, Methylin ER, Methylofenidan, Methylphenidan, Methylphenidatum, Methylphenidylacetate hydrochloride, Methypatch, Metilfenidat hydrochloride, Metilfenidato, Metilfenidato, Phenidylate, Plimasine, PMS-Methylphenidate, Riphenidate, Ritalin LA, Ritalin SR, Ritalin-SR, Ritaline, Ritcher Works
Modafinil	**Provigil**, Dea No. 1680, Modafinilo, Modafinilum, Moderateafinil, Modiodal
Pemoline	**Cylert**, Azoksodon, Azoxodon, Azoxodone, Betanamin, Centramin, Constimol, Cylert Chewable, Dantromin, Deltamin, Deltamine, Endolin, Fenoxazol, Fio, Hyton, Hyton asa, Juston-Wirkstoff, Kethamed, Myamin, NPL 1, Nitan, Notair, Okodon, PIO, Pemolin, Pemolina, Phenalone, Phenilone, Pheniminooxazolidinone, Phenoxazole, Phenylisohydantoin, Phenylpseudohydantoin, Pioxol, Pomoline, Pondex, Ronyl, Senior, Sigmadyn, Sistra, Sistral, Sofro, Stimul, Stimulol, Tradon, Tradone, Volital, Volitol, Yh 1

Chapter 3

Bipolar Disorder

The Web site for NAMI, the National Alliance for Mental Illness, at www.nami.org, describes bipolar disorder as follows:

What is Bipolar Disorder?
Bipolar Disorder, or manic depression, is a serious brain disorder that causes extreme shifts in mood, energy, and functioning. It affects 2.3 million adult Americans, which is about 1.2 percent of the population, and can run in families. The disorder affects men and women equally. Bipolar Disorder is characterized by episodes of mania and depression that can last from days to months. Bipolar Disorder is a chronic and generally life-long condition with recurring episodes that often begin in adolescence or early adulthood, and occasionally even in children. It generally requires lifelong treatment, and recovery between episodes is often poor. Generally, those who suffer from Bipolar Disorder have symptoms of both mania and depression (sometimes at the same time).

What are the symptoms of mania?
Mania is the word that describes the activated phase of Bipolar Disorder. The symptoms of mania may include:

- either an elated, happy mood or an irritable, angry, unpleasant mood
- increased activity or energy
- more thoughts and faster thinking than normal
- increased talking, more rapid speech than normal
- ambitious, often grandiose, plans
- poor judgement
- increased sexual interest and activity

- decreased sleep and decreased need for sleep

What are the symptoms of depression?

Depression is the other phase of Bipolar Disorder. The symptoms of depression may include:

- depressed or apathetic mood
- decreased activity and energy
- restlessness and irritability
- fewer thoughts than usual and slowed thinking
- less talking and slowed speech
- less interest or participation in, and less enjoyment of activities normally enjoyed
- decreased sexual interest and activity
- hopeless and helpless feelings
- feelings of guilt and worthlessness
- pessimistic outlook
- thoughts of suicide
- change in appetite (either eating more or eating less)
- change in sleep patterns (either sleeping more or sleeping less)

What is a "mixed" state?

A mixed state is when symptoms of mania and depression occur at the same time. During a mixed state depressed mood accompanies manic activation.

What is rapid cycling?

Sometimes individuals may experience an increased frequency of episodes. When four or more episodes of illness occur within a 12-month period, the individual is said to have Bipolar Disorder with rapid cycling. Rapid cycling is more common in women.

The category of bipolar disorder breaks down into a few sub-categories. The University of Maryland Medical Center Web site (www.umm.edu/patiented/index) has this to say about the varieties:

Bipolar Disorder Categories

Bipolar disorder is classified according to symptom severity as bipolar disorder I, bipolar disorder II, and cyclothymic disorder. Some experts believe these are actually separate disorders with different biologic factors accounting for their differences.

Bipolar Disorder Type I. Bipolar disorder type I is characterized by at least one manic episode, with or without major depression. With mania, either euphoria or irritability may mark the phase, and there are significant negative effects (such as sexual recklessness, excessive impulse shopping, sudden traveling) on a patients' social life, work, or both. Untreated mania lasts at least a week or results in hospitalization. Typically, depressive episodes tend to last six to 12 months if untreated. However, untreated manic episodes last three to six months.

Hypomania and Bipolar Disorder Type II. Bipolar disorder type II is characterized by at least one episode of hypomania and at least one episode of major depression. With hypomania the symptoms of mania (euphoria or irritability) appear in milder forms and are of shorter duration. Bipolar II depression is the most commonly expressed form of all bipolar disorders and it is also highly associated with suicide risk.

Cyclothymic Disorder. Cyclothymic disorder is not as severe as either bipolar disorder II or I, but the condition is more chronic. The disorder lasts at least two years, with single episodes persisting for more than two months. Cyclothymic disorder may be a precursor to full-blown bipolar disorder in some people or it may continue as a low-grade chronic condition.

Course of the Illness
Bipolar disorder can be severe and long-term, or it can be mild with infrequent episodes. The usual pattern of bipolar disorder is one of increasing intensity and duration of symptoms that progresses slowly over many years. (Patients with the disease, however, may experience symptoms in very different ways.) A bipolar disorder patient averages 8 to 10 manic or depressive episodes over a lifetime, but some people experience more and some fewer episodes.

Typical Bipolar Cycles. In most cases of bipolar disorder, the depressive phases far outnumber manic phases, and the cycles of mania and depression are neither regular nor predictable. Many patients, in fact, experience mixed mania, or a mixed state, in which both mania and depression occur.

Rapid Cycling. About 15% of patients have a temporary, complicated phase known as rapid cycling, in which the manic and depressive episodes alternate at least four times a year and, in severe cases, can even progress to several cycles a day. (Some experts suggest that rapid cycling may first occur in bipolar disorder patients who are on antidepressants, which trigger a switch to mania and set up a cyclical pattern.)

Additional types of bipolar disorder are under consideration, but are not yet considered standard diagnostic categories. These additional types include

Bipolar Disorder Type III. Bipolar disorder Type III refers to manic or hypomanic episodes induced by antidepressant medication. This situation can arise when someone who has bipolar disorder is diagnosed with depression and given an SSRI, or other serotonergic medication, without an accompanying mood stabilizer.

Bipolar Disorder Type IV. Bipolar disorder Type IV refers to a condition characterized by the late development of depression in an individual of lifelong "hyperthymic" temperament, meaning someone who has shown hypomanic traits on a steady, as opposed to episodic, basis.

Psychotic episodes can also be a symptom of bipolar disorder. The presence of psychosis makes diagnosis more difficult, as the illness can easily be confused with schizophrenia.

This chapter will refer to normal depression as *unipolar* depression, to distinguish it from the depressive episodes of bipolar disorder. While unipolar depression is bad enough, people with bipolar disorder have twice the number of undesirable, and uncontrollable, moods, as well as no control over the transition between them. Thus it it is not surprising bipolar disorder is more difficult to treat than unipolar depression.

3.1   Causes of Bipolar Disorder

The cause of bipolar disorder remains unknown. It seems clear that the disorder involves brain chemistry at some level, and possibly neurological problems, especially given the utility of some anti-seizure medications in treatment. It also seems clear that, as for Major Depressive Disorder, bipolar disorder is partly inherent in the brain, and partly a response to external circumstances.

The principal hypothesis for bipolar disorder is the "Kindling Model." This model was first developed in the context of seizure disorders (specifically epilepsy), where it was discovered that repeated electrical stimulation of the brain in rats, at levels too low to cause seizures initially, nevertheless resulted in seizures developing after a couple of weeks. The rats' brains had become sensitized to this stimulation in a way that resulted in seizures from levels of stimulation that had formerly been too low to cause them. (It was found that similar results were producible through chemical stimulation, as well.)

The term "kindling" was selected because the process seemed analogous to lighting a fire (burning a big log) by lighting lots of little fires first (small pieces of kindling wood).

The kindling hypothesis has some implications.

- First, the more bipolar episodes (or seizures) one has had, the more likely one is to have them in the future, and more frequently, meaning the problem worsens if untreated.

- Second, the worsening may result in a transitioning to rapid-cycling and treatment-resistant bipolar disorder.

- Third, mood episodes that were initially triggered by environmental influences (such as a bad day at work) can become spontaneous, requiring no triggers.

- Fourth, terminating treatment can not only cause a relapse of the disorder, but *result in it getting worse, and becoming resistant to treatment that formerly worked.*

These implications are observed in clinical practice.

3.2 The Role of Gamma-Aminobutyric Acid (GABA)

One neurotransmitter that does appear to play a major role in both seizure activity and bipolar depression (particularly the manic phase) is gamma-aminobutyric acid (GABA), which is described in Section 1.3.2.

Receptors for GABA come in three varieties: GABA-A, GABA-B, and GABA-C. The Gabitril Web site (www.gabitril.com/physicians/gaba/default.asp) has this to say about GABA:

> G-aminobutyric acid (GABA) is the most important inhibitory neurotransmitter in the central nervous system (CNS) and is widely distributed throughout the brain. Approximately 60-75% of all synapses in the CNS are GABAergic.
>
> *The Role of GABA in CNS*
> GABA binds to three principal receptors, each of which is involved in different physiologic functions:
>
> - GABA-A receptors mediate fast inhibitory synaptic transmissions; they regulate neuronal excitability (eg, seizure threshold) and rapid changes in mood (eg, anxiety, panic, and response to stress); they are targets of benzodiazepines, barbiturates, and ethanol
> - GABA-B receptors mediate slow inhibitory potentials; they appear to be important in memory, mood (depression), and pain

- GABA-C receptors—their physiologic role has not yet been described

Enhancing GABA Activity

GABAergic activity may be enhanced by either:

- Stimulating GABA-A receptors (GABA-A-receptor agonists or modulating compounds)

- Inhibition of GABA metabolism

- Direct inhibition of GABA reuptake from the synapse by blocking the action of GATs (selective GABA-reuptake inhibitors)

GATs are membrane-transporter proteins that remove GABA from the synaptic cleft.

Four distinct GATs have been identified: GAT-1, GAT-2, GAT-3, and BGT-1; they are located on neurons, both pre- and postsynaptically, and on glial cells. They differ in CNS distribution and localization.

- GAT-1 is the primary GABA transporter in the brain.

- The density of GAT-1 is highest in the frontal and parietal cortex.

Finally, medications that increase GABA concentration or effectiveness tend to cause sleepiness, and benzodiazepines (which enhance GABA activity) are occasionally prescribed as sleep medication for occasional insomnia (see Section 3.9). GABA reuptake inhibitors may also promote sleepiness. It may be that the increase in GABA activity or concentration, which produces sleepiness in many individuals, acts primarily to counter mania (without sleepiness) in those who have bipolar disorder,

3.3   Treatments for Bipolar Disorder

Bipolar disorder requires medical treatment. Therapy alone cannot address the underlying causes, which are neurological in origin. This is in contrast to the case of unipolar depression, as some instances of the latter arise purely from factors within the capability of the individual to change, often with help from a therapist. However, therapy does have a role to play in the overall management of bipolar disorder. A good therapist can help a patient develop improved coping strategies for dealing with the illness. This is more important than it might sound, as the nature of bipolar disorder (particularly manic states) can severely distort the patient's capacity for judgment, and a therapist's input is therefore of particular value. For this reason, therapy is recommended as part of the approach for treating bipolar disorder, at least until the patient and therapist agree that the patient is stabilized and doing well.

The only technique, other than medication, that has been found to be effective in treating bipolar disorder is that of electroconvulsive therapy, or ECT. This technique, which is described in Section 1.7.2, deserves careful consideration. Because of its drawbacks, ECT is not the method of choice for treating bipolar disorder; however, it is effective, and worth considering if medication has failed.

The experimental treatments described in Section 1.8 may be of interest as well, although their effectiveness for bipolar disorder has not yet been well established. However, the reader is advised to review these approaches in addition to the other techniques described below.

The standard strategy for treating bipolar disorder is to prescribe two medications: An antidepressant (to treat the depression) and a mood stabilizer (to prevent manic episodes and cycling). More recently, some of the atypical antipsychotic medications have also been used in place of, or in addition to, mood stabilizers (see Chapter 4 for details). The antipsychotics are particularly useful in cases where psychosis is present. (The medication Symbyax, which is a combination of the antidepressant Fluoxetine and the atypical antipsychotic Olanzapine, has been approved for use in treating the depressive phase of bipolar disorder. Information about Symbyax may be found in Section 2.5.3.)

Antidepressants are described in Chapter 2, while mood stabilizers are described in detail in the following sections. While no widely-accepted test exists to identify the most appropriate medications for a particular person, the experimental technique of Section 1.8.1.1 may be worth investigating for this purpose.

The mechanisms by which mood stabilizers work are even less well-understood than those of antidepressant medications. While the latter are thought to exert their effects most often by increasing the concentration of neurotransmitters (specifically serotonin, norepinephrine, and dopamine), the mechanisms of mood stabilizers are less understood and more varied in nature.

Some of the mood stabilizers prescribed for bipolar disorder are occasionally prescribed for unipolar depression, either solely, or in combination with other antidepressants. While this type of augmentation is not uncommon, its effectiveness is not well understood.

Warning! It is very important that anyone suffering from bipolar disorder *not* take any antidepressant that increases serotonin concentration (such as the SSRI, SNRI, TCA, and MAOI categories), without taking a mood-stabilizer medication at the same time. Taking one of these antidepressants without a mood stabilizer can trigger manic states. If you find that taking one of these antidepressants leads to excessive spending, grandiose behavior, hyperactivity and insomnia, consult your psychiatrist immediately. You may have bipolar disorder, and require an appropriate treatment for it.

3.4   Lithium

Lithium compounds have been used for a very long time, relative to other psychotropic medications. Lithium's beneficial effects on stabilizing the moods of people suffering from bipolar disorder (long before the illness had that name) were
noticed in the late 1800s, although the Food and Drug Administration (FDA) did
not approve lithium for this medical use until 1970.

Lithium was the the only FDA-approved medication for chronic mania until
2004, when Olanzapine (an anti-psychotic medication) was approved for this use.

3.4.1   Mechanism

The mechanism by which lithium alleviates mania is not known, although some
things are known about its effects on neurochemistry. Lithium may exert a dual
effect on receptors for the neurotransmitter glutamate, regulating the glutamate
concentration so that it stays between minimum and maximum limits (see, for example, the description at bipolar.about.com/cs/lithium/a/0103_lithium1.htm). It
also alters sodium transport in nerve and muscle cells and increases the metabolism
of catecholamines (epinephrine, norepinephrine, and dopamine) in the brain.

3.4.2   Benefits

Lithium compounds are used to treat the manic episodes of bipolar disorder. They
are sometimes prescribed to augment the effect of antidepressants in the treatment of unipolar depression, and to treat Obsessive-Compulsive disorder. They are
highly effective (as psychotropic medications go), with approximately 60–80% rate
of success for classic mania (30–40% or dyshporic/psychotic mania or mixed states,
20–30% for rapid-cycling bipolar-affective disorder).

3.4.3   Principal Drawbacks

The amount of lithium required for optimum treatment of mania is, unfortunately,
not much less than the amount at which toxicity appears. Thus it is important to
monitor the concentration of lithium in the blood carefully, to ensure that it does
not rise above the threshold for toxic effects. The most common side effects are gastrointestinal (GI) problems (nausea, vomiting, diarrhea), weight gain, and tremor.
GI problems and muscular weakness may be early symptoms of lithium toxicity, and
should be reported to the physician immediately. Renal (kidney) function should
be checked periodically (usually annually) to look for signs of trouble.

Lithium can cause hypothyroidism, a condition in which the thyroid gland produces inadequate levels of thyroid hormones (see Section 1.5. Thus thyroid function
should also be checked periodically (typically on an annual basis).

Warning! Lithium has the second-highest risk level (of four) for causing QT Prolongation and serious abnormalities of heart rhythm. Medications at this risk level have been associated with QT Prolongation, but not proven to cause it. The risk for QT Prolongation is not considered high, but medications with lower risk are preferred, especially for anyone who has Long QT Syndrome. If you cannot substitute a medication with lower risk, be alert for heart palpitations. If you experience palpitations, report them to your doctor immediately.

3.4.4   Medications

Main Brand Name	Chemical Name	Chemical Type	Half Life	Washout Time	On-Label Uses	Off-Label Uses
Lithobid	Lithium Carbonate	Lithium salt	24 hours	5 days	Bipolar Disorder (Manic phase)	Depression (Adjunctive)
Priadel	Lithium Citrate	Lithium salt (liquid form)	24 hours	5 days	Bipolar Disorder (Manic phase)	Depression (Adjunctive)

3.4.5   Brand Names

Chemical Name	Brand Names (Principal in Bold)
Lithium Carbonate	**Lithobid**, Camcolit, Carbolit, Carbolith, Carbolithium, Ceglution 300, Ceglution, Contemnol, Duralith, Eskalith, Eskalith-Cr, Hynorex Retard, Lentolith, Licab, Licarb, Licarbium, Lidin, Limas, Liskonum, Litarex, Lithane, Litheum 300, Lithicarb, Lithionate, Lithizine, Lithocap, Lithonate, Lithotabs, Litilent, Litocarb, Maniprex, Milithin, Neurolepsin, Neurolithium, Phanate, Phasal,Plenur, Priadel Retard, Priadel, Quilonium-R, Quilonorm Retardtabletten, Quilonum Retard, Quilonum SR, Teralithe, Theralite
Lithium Citrate	**Priadel**

3.5   Valproate

Valproate (used generically for this category) is an anticonvulsant medication that has been found effective for the treatment of the manic episodes of bipolar disorder. Valproate is also prescribed to prevent migraine headaches, in addition to its use in treating seizures and bipolar disorder.

3.5.1   Mechanism

The mechanism by which Valproate alleviates mania is not known. It has been suggested that its activity in the treatment of epilepsy is due to increasing the brain concentration of Gamma-aminobutyric acid (GABA). However, Valproate appears less likely to cause sleepiness than medications known to boost GABA, which may indicate that Valproate's effect on mania works in some other fashion.

Note that Divalproex is a mixture of Sodium Valproate and Valproic Acid.

3.5.2   Benefits

Valproate is effective in treating mania and seizures.

3.5.3   Principal Drawbacks

Valproate can cause liver (hepatic) damage or failure. Thus it is important to conduct blood tests to monitor the liver function in patients who are taking this medication, and terminate the medication if liver damage is detected. Valproate can also cause birth defects, if taken by pregnant women, or pancreatitis (inflammation of the pancreas). Any abdominal pain, nausea, or vomiting that occurs after beginning treatment with Valproate should be reported to a doctor immediately for diagnosis.

Weight gain is also a common, though not universal, side effect.

The different formulations of Valproate (in the table below) work in the same fashion inside the body (once converted into Valproate ions after ingestion), but are not identical in terms of dosage. Exercise care when converting from one formulation to another.

3.5.4 Medications

Main Brand Name	Chemical Name	Chemical Type	Half Life	Washout Time	On-Label Uses	Off-Label Uses
Depacon	Sodium Valproate		24 hours	5 days	Bipolar Disorder (Manic phase); Seizures (Monotherapy, Adjunctive)	Depression
Depakene	Valproic Acid		24 hours	5 days	Bipolar Disorder (Manic phase); Seizures (Monotherapy, Adjunctive)	Depression
Depakote	Divalproex		24 hours	5 days	Bipolar Disorder (Manic phase); Seizures (Monotherapy, Adjunctive)	Depression

3.5.5 Brand Names

Chemical Name	Brand Names (Principal in Bold)
Divalproex	**Depakote**, Convulex, DPA, Depakene, Depakine, Dipropylacetic acid, Divalproex sodium, Elvetium, Epilim, Epival, Ergenyl, Everiden, Mylproin, N-dipropylacetic acid, N-DPA, Novoseven, Propylvaleric acid, Valcote, Valnar
Sodium Valproate	**Depacon**, Convulex Syrup, Convulex, Depakene, Depakin, Depakine Depakote, Druppels, Depakine, Depakote, Depalept Chrono, Depalept, Epilam, Epilex, Epilim Chrono, Epilim, Epival, Ergenyl, Leptilan, Orfil, Orfiril, Orfiril Retard, Petilin, Valcote, Valeptol, Valoin, Valpakine, Valparin, Valporal, Valprax, Valpro, Valsup
Valproic Acid	**Depakene**, 2 PP (base), Alti-Valproic, Bruceine D, Convulex, DPA, DPA (VAN), Delepsine, Depacon, Depakin, Depakine, Deproic, Di-n-propylacetic acid, Di-n-propylessigsaure, Dipropylacetic acid, Dom-Valproic, Epiject, Epilex, Epilim, Epival, Ergenyl, Kyselina 2-propylvalerova, Leptilan, Med Valproic, Mylproin, Myproic Acid, N-Dipropylacetic acid, N-DPA, Novo-Valproic, Nu-Valproic, Orfiril, Penta-Valproic, 2-propyl-Pentanoic acid, Propylvaleric acid, Sodium hydrogen divalproate, Sprinkle, Valcote, 2-propyl-Valeric acid, Valparin, Valporal, Valpro, Valproate semisodique, Valproate semisodium, Valproato semisodico, Valproatum seminatricum, Valprosid

3.6   Enzyme-Inducing Anti-Epileptic Drug (EIAED)

This category is defined not by how the medications achieve their therapeutic results, or by their chemical structure, but by their effects on the liver. EIAED medications induce (cause) the liver to create more of the CYP450 enzyme. A dose that was effective initially may need to be raised over time, as the liver produces more of the enzyme, and breaks down the medication faster.

3.6.1   Mechanism

The mechanism by which these medications alleviate mania and seizures is not known.

Oxcarbazepine is chemically similar to Carbamazepine, but has an extra oxygen atom.

3.6.2   Benefits

These medications are effective in treating mania and seizures.

Oxcarbazepine's tendency to cause drowsiness may be useful for people who have difficulty sleeping.

3.6.3   Principal Drawbacks

Because of their enzyme-inducing effects, the dosage may need to be raised over time in order to maintain a constant level of effectiveness. Also, changing the liver's behavior in this fashion affects other biochemical processes that involve the liver. As a result, there can be numerous drug-drug interactions, including those that involve hormones and birth-control pills. Anyone considering a major change in diet should consult a doctor beforehand, as they can also have unexpected results (such as disruption of glucose processing). In general, one should be sure to discuss possible problems with the doctor, and keep them in mind when taking medications or altering eating habits.

Carbamazepine commonly causes nausea, confusion, fatigue, dulled thinking, and clumsiness (often temporary). Rarely, Carbamazepine can cause aplastic anemia and agranulocytosis. Periodic blood samples should be taken to monitor for these problems. Immediately report to physician any rash, fever, sore throat, or easy bruising.

Oxcarbazepine commonly causes somnolence, tremor, abnormal gait. Oxcarbazepine can also cause an odd, dangerous, but easily treatable condition known as hyponatremia. Nausea, fatigue, seizures, and dulled thinking should be reported to the physician immediately.

3.6.4 Medications

Main Brand Name	Chemical Name	Chemical Type	Half Life	Wash-out Time	On-Label Uses	Off-Label Uses
Tegretol	Carba-mazepine	Tricyclic	16 hours	3 days	Seizures (Partial, not Absence)	Bipolar Disorder (Manic phase)
Trileptal	Oxcar-bazepine	Tricyclic	11 hours	3 days	Seizures (Partial, Monotherapy and Adjunctive)	Bipolar Disorder (Manic phase)

3.6.5 Brand Names

Chemical Name	Brand Names (Principal in Bold)
Carba-mazepine	**Tegretol**, Apo-Carbamazepine, Atretol, Biston, Calepsin, Camapine, Carbadac, Carbamazepen, Carbamezepine, Carbatol, Carbatrol, Carbazene, Carbazep, Carbazepine, Carbazina, Carbelan, Carbium, Carmaz, Carpaz, Carzepin, Carzepine, Clostedal, Convuline, Degranol, Epileptol, Epileptol CR, Epitol, Eposal Retard, Equetro, Espa-lepsin, Finlepsin, Foxalepsin, Foxalepsin Retard, Hermolepsin, Karbamazepin, Kodapan, Lexin, Macrepan, Mazetol, Neugeron, Neurotol, Neurotop, Neurotop Retard, Nordotol, Novo-Carbamaz, Nu-Carbamazepine, Panitol, Sirtal, Stazepin, Stazepine, Tardotol, Taro-Carbamazepine, Taro-Carbamazepine Cr, Taver, Tegol, Tegretal, Tegretol, Tegretol Chewtabs, Tegretol Cr, Tegretol-Xr, Telesmin, Telestin, Temporal Slow, Temporol, Teril, Timonil, Timonil Retard
Oxcar-bazepine	**Trileptal**, Oxaprozin, Oxaprozine, Oxcarbamazepine

3.7 GABA Analogs (GA)

The medications in this category are those which increase the concentration or effects of GABA, and are not otherwise categorized.

3.7.1 Mechanism

The classification of Gabapentin is uncertain. It is not defined as a GABA agonist, although it is structurally related to GABA, and binds to some sites in the neocortex and hippocampus of the rat brain. Gabapentin is also not a reuptake inhibitor of GABA, serotonin, norepinephrine, or dopamine, nor does it convert into GABA or a GABA agonist. The mechanism by which Gabapentin alleviates seizusres is not known. The mechanism by which it alleviates pain from neuralgia is also not known.

Tiagabine is a selective GABA reuptake inhibitor (GRI). It increases the concentration of GABA in the brain by binding to the GAT-1 transporter, which is the protein predominantly responsible for reuptake of GABA into the presynaptic (emitting) neurons and glial cells.

3.7.2   Benefits

These medications are effective in treating mania and seizures.

Gabapentin is an effective treatment for herpes-induced pain and seizures. Its effectiveness in treating bipolar disorder has not been well established.

Tiagabine is an effective treatment for mania and seizures, though like all psychotropic medications, it is not always effective in all people.

3.7.3   Principal Drawbacks

Typical side effects include dizziness, somnolence, and fatigue. Gabapentin has the odd features of not being metabolized significantly (it is excreted in unaltered form), and its concentration in the body does not increase in proportion to the dose. The higher the dose, the smaller the percentage of the medication is actually absorbed by the body. The result is that the amount in the body does increase with dose, but at decreasing rates.

Tiagabine is reputed to work well for 7–10 days in many people, as a treatment for bipolar, panic, and post-straumatic stress disorders, then suddenly stop. The transient benefit can be quite frustrating. Typical side effects include dizziness, somnolence, irritability, fatigue, nausea, and tremor.

3.7.4 Medications

Main Brand Name	Chemical Name	Chemical Type	Half Life	Wash-out Time	On-Label Uses	Off-Label Uses
Gabitril	Tiagabine		8 hours	2 days	Seizures (Partial, Adjunctive)	Bipolar Disorder (Manic phase); Generalized Anxiety Disorder; Panic Disorder; Post-Traumatic Stress Disorder
Neurontin	Gabapentin		6 hours	1 day	Seizures (Partial, Adjunctive); Neuralgia (Postherpetic, i.e., from Herpes infections)	Bipolar Disorder (Manic phase)

3.7.5 Brand Names

Chemical Name	Brand Names (Principal in Bold)
Gaba-pentin	**Neurontin**, Aclonium, Gabapentine, Gabapentino, Gabapentinum, Gabapetin, Novo-Gabapentin
Tiagabine	**Gabitril**, Tiagabina, Tiagabinum

3.8 Miscellaneous Anticonvulsants

The medications in this category are those that have not been otherwise categorized.

3.8.1 Mechanism

The mechanism by which Lamotrigine alleviates bipolar disorder is not known. What is known is that it weakly inhibits serotonin receptors. It does not inhibit the reuptake of norepinephrine, dopamine, or serotonin. It lengthens the intervals between the occurrence of mood episodes (depression, mania, hypomania, and mixed episodes) in patients who are treated for acute mood episodes with standard therapy (such as with Valproate). (Ideally, Lamotrigine would lengthen the interval

between episodes to the point where the episodes no longer occur, but this cannot
be guaranteed.)

The mechanism by which Topiramate alleviates seizures is not known. What is
known is that it increases the effectiveness of GABA, by increasing the frequency
at which GABA activates GABA receptors.

3.8.2   Benefits

These medications are effective in treating mania and seizures.

Lamotrigine is an effective treatment for bipolar disorder and seizures. Compared to other mood stabilizers, it is unusual in that it does not act primarily to
suppress mania, but rather to reduce the severity and frequency of the extremes of
bipolar disorder (manic and depressive states). It has been found to be of benefit
in treating normal (unipolar) depression, as well the depressive phase of bipolar
disorder.

Topiramate is an effective treatment for seizures, though like all psychotropic
medications, it is not always effective in all people.

3.8.3   Principal Drawbacks

Although this problem occurs rarely (roughly 1 out of 1000), Lamotrigine can cause a
dangerous rash, including Stevens-Johnson Syndrome and Toxic Epidermal Necrolysis. The rash can cause serious tissue damage, and even death. The risk of developing
the rash is greater for pediatric patients than adults, or for people who are taking
Valproate (which approximately doubles the elimination half life of Lamotrigine).
If such a rash occurs, it is most likely to occur within 2 to 8 weeks after starting the
medication (though there is no guarantee that one won't occur later).

The risk of a dangerous rash is reduced if one slowly increases the dosage from a
small quantity to the therapeutic level. Thus one typically receives a starter pack of
Lamotrigine customized for increasing the dose to useful levels at a controlled rate.

While the rash issue is serious, the possibility should not deter someone who
may benefit from the medication from trying it. The physician and patient should
simply be careful to monitor for any adverse reactions.

In spite of the caution about rashes, Lamotrigine generally has little in the way
of side effects. For people who take Lamotrigine as a seizure treatment, the more
common side effects include headache, nausea, dizziness, clumsiness, drowsiness,
runny nose, rash, and double or blurred vision. For those who take it as a bipolar
treatment, side effects are less common; of these, the more common side include
back, neck, or abdominal pain, nausea, constipation, insomnia, drowsiness, runny
nose, and rash.

Care must be exercised when combining Lamotrigine with Valproate, due to the
effects of the latter on the chemistry of the former. The dosage of Lamotrigine may

need to be adjusted downwards relative to what would be considered appropriate in the absence of Valproate.

Rarely, myopia and glaucoma can develop, so the patient should report any new vision problems immediately. Common side effects include fatigue, dizziness, clumsiness, tremor, impaired speech, nausea, weight loss, drowsiness, nervousness, memory impairment, loss of appetite, depression, and decreased attention span.

3.8.4 Medications

Main Brand Name	Chemical Name	Chemical Type	Half Life	Wash-out Time	On-Label Uses	Off-Label Uses
Lamictal	Lamotrigine	Phenyl-triazine	33 hours	7 days	Bipolar Disorder (General), type I; Seizures (Partial, Monotherapy or Adjunctive); Seizures (Generalized, Adjunctive)	Depression
Topamax	Topiramate	Mono-saccharide	21 hours	4 days	Seizures (Adjunctive)	Bipolar Disorder (General), type I; Depression

3.8.5 Brand Names

Chemical Name	Brand Names (Principal in Bold)
Lamo-trigine	**Lamictal**, Lamictal Cd, Lamotrigina, Lamotriginum
Topir-amate	**Topamax**, Tipiramate, Tipiramato, Topamax (TN), Topamax Sprinkle, Topiramato, Topiramatum

3.9 Benzodiazepines

Medications in the Benzodiazepine category are typically prescribed for Anxiety and Panic Disorders, and as an aid in sleeping. Some of them are also of use in treating seizure and bipolar disorders.

3.9.1   Mechanism

Benzodiazepines enhance the activity of Gamma-aminobutyric acid (GABA), which has a calming effect on the brain. They are anticonvulsant medications, useful in treating seizures, and like other anticonvulsant medications, are often useful in treating bipolar disorder as well.

3.9.2   Benefits

Benzodiazepines are relatively weak mood stabilizers. Their principal advantage is that they work quickly, and can be a good choice when a seizure or manic episode is starting. They may are useful in the long-term treatment of anxiety in the event that more standard antidepressants are unsuccessful.

Lorazepam is particularly fast-acting, with minimal side effects.

3.9.3   Principal Drawbacks

Because they are relatively weak mood stabilizers, Benzodiazepines are generally not a good choice for long-term control of mania. Also, they are addictive, and can aggravate depression (unipolar or bipolar).

Alprazolam is considered to be one of the most, perhaps the most, potent and addictive of all benzodiazepines.

3.9.4 Medications

Main Brand Name	Chemical Name	Chemical Type	Half Life	Wash-out Time	On-Label Uses	Off-Label Uses
Ativan	Lorazepam	Benzo-diazepine	18 hours	4 days	anxiety; Seizures	Bipolar Disorder (Manic phase); Insomnia
Klonopin	Clonazepam	Benzo-diazepine	36 hours	1 week	Panic Disorder (with or without agoraphobia); Seizures (Monotherapy, Adjunctive)	Bipolar Disorder (Manic phase)
Librium	Chlordi-azepoxide	Benzo-diazepine	36 hours	1 week	anxiety	Bipolar Disorder (Manic phase)
Tranxene	Clorazepate	Benzo-diazepine	2 days	10 days	anxiety; Seizures (Adjunctive)	Bipolar Disorder (Manic phase)
Valium	Diazepam	Benzo-diazepine	2 days	10 days	anxiety; Muscle Spasms	Bipolar Disorder (Manic phase)
Xanax	Alprazolam	Benzo-diazepine	11 hours	4 days	Panic Disorder (with or without agoraphobia)	Bipolar Disorder (Manic phase)

3.9.5   Brand Names

Chemical Name	Brand Names (Principal in Bold)
Alprazolam	**Xanax**, Alplax, Alpronax, Alviz, Bestrol, Cassadan, Constan, D 65MT, Esparon, Frontal, Intensol, Niravam, Restyl, Solanax, TUS-1, Tafil, Tranax, Trankimazin, Tranquinal, Xanax XR, Xanor
Chlordiazepoxide	**Librium**, A-Poxide, Abboxide, Apo-Chlordiazepoxide, Balance, CD 2, CDO, CDP, Chloradiazepoxide, Chlordiazachel, Chlordiazepoxid, Chlordiazepoxide Base, Chlordiazepoxidum, Chloridazepoxide, Chloridiazepide, Chloridiazepoxide, Chlorodiazepoxide, Chlozepid, Clopoxide, Clordiazepossido, Contol, Control, Decacil, Eden, Elenium, Helogaphen, Ifibrium, Kalmocaps, Librax, Librelease, Librinin, Libritabs, Limbitrol, Limbitrol Ds, Lygen, Menrium, Mesural, Methaminodiazepoxide, Mildmen, Multum, Napoton, Napton, Novo-Poxide, Psicosan, Radepur, Risolid, Silibrin, Tropium, Viopsicol
Clonazepam	**Klonopin**, Antelepsin, Antilepsin, Chlonazepam, Cloazepam, Clonazepamum, Clonopin, Iktorivil, Klonopin, Klonopin Rapidly Disintegrating, Landsen, Rivotril
Clorazepate	**Tranxene**, Chlorazepate, Chlorazepic acid, Clorazepate dipotassium, Clorazepic acid, Clorazepic acid, Gen-xene
Diazepam	**Valium**, Alboral, Aliseum, Alupram, Amiprol, An-Ding, Ansiolin, Ansiolisina, Apaurin, Apo-Diazepam, Apozepam, Armonil, Assival, Atensine, Atilen, Bensedin, Bialzepam, Calmocitene, Calmpose, Cercine, Ceregulart, Condition, DAP, Diacepan, Dialag, Dialar, Diapam, Diastat, Diazemuls, Diazemulus, Diazepam Intensol, Diazepan, Diazetard, Dienpax, Dipam, Dipezona, Dizac, Domalium, Duksen, Duxen, E-Pam, Eridan, Eurosan, Evacalm, Faustan, Faustan, Freudal, Frustan, Gewacalm, Gihitan, Horizon, Kabivitrum, Kiatrium, LA III, La-Iii, Lamra, Lembrol, Levium, Liberetas, Mandrozep, Methyldiazepinone, Methyldiazepinone, Pharmaceutical, Morosan, Neurolytril, Noan, Novazam, Novo-Dipam, Paceum, Pacitran, Paranten, Paxate, Paxel, Plidan, Pms-Diazepam, Pro-Pam, Q-Pam, Q-Pam Relanium, Quetinil, Quiatril, Quievita, Relaminal, Relanium, Relax, Renborin, Ruhsitus, S.A. R.L., Saromet, Sedapam, Sedipam, Seduksen, Seduxen, Serenack, Serenamin, Serenzin, Servizepam, Setonil, Sibazon, Sibazone, Solis, Sonacon, Stesolid, Stesolin, Tensopam, Tranimul, Tranqdyn, Tranquase, Tranquirit, Tranquo-Puren, Tranquo-Tablinen, Umbrium, Unisedil, Usempax Ap, Valaxona, Valeo, Valiquid, Valitran, Valrelease, Vatran, Velium, Vival, Vivol, Zetran, Zipan
Lorazepam	**Ativan**, (+/-)-Lorazepam, Almazine, Alzapam, Anxiedin, Aplacassee, Bonatranquan, Delormetazepam, Emotival, Idalprem, L-Lorazepam Acetate, Lorabenz, Lorax, Loraz, Lorazepam Intensol, Lorsilan, O-Chlorooxazepam, O-Chloroxazepam, Pro Dorm, Psicopax, Punktyl, Quait, Securit, Sedatival, Sedazin, Somagerol, Tavor, Temesta, Wypax

3.10 Antipsychotics

The newest category of medications used for the treatment of bipolar disorder is that of the atypical antipsychotics. These medications were originally developed to treat schizophrenia, as well as psychosis arising from various conditions, including bipolar disorder.

The antipsychotic medications that have been found to be useful for treating bipolar disorder are described in Section 4.5. While it is generally a good thing that additional medications have become available to treat bipolar disorder, the antipsychotic medications are generally less safe, and have more drastic side effects, than mood stabilizers and antidepressants. For this reason, they should be used with caution, and primarily in cases where the illness does not respond to other treatments.

The medication Symbyax, which is a combination of the antidepressant Fluoxetine and the atypical antipsychotic Olanzapine, has been approved for use in treating the depressive phase of bipolar disorder. Information about Symbyax may be found in Section 2.5.3.

For more details about antipsychotic medications, their mechanisms, benefits, and drawbacks, see Chapter 4.

Chapter 4

Schizophrenia and Psychosis

Psychosis is not an illness, but a name for a set of symptoms that often occur together, and for which the central characteristic is a major discrepancy between reality and an individual's perception of it. The most familiar symptoms of psychosis are hallucinations (false perceptions) and delusions (false beliefs). A common but less obvious symptom is anosognosia, or the disbelief that anything is wrong with the person's perceptions and thoughts.

Anosognosia greatly complicates the treatment of psychosis. Those whose illness is accompanied by anosognosia are likely to resist treatment that they believe is unnecessary, especially if they suffer from paranoia as well. The combination of anosognosia and paranoia can make treatment impossible, unless enforced involuntarily, on an in-patient basis.

The illness most closely associated with psychosis is schizophrenia, although psychosis can also result from the manic episodes of bipolar disorder, brain injuries, an episode of extreme stress, or psychoactive drugs.

Wikipedia defines psychosis by the following symptoms:

Hallucinations

A hallucination is defined as any sensory perception that is perceived in the absence of an external stimulus. Hallucinations are different from illusions, which are the misperception of external stimuli. Hallucinations may occur in any of the five senses and take on almost any form, which may include simple sensations (such as lights, colors, tastes, smells) to more meaningful experiences such as seeing and interacting with fully formed animals and people, hearing voices and complex tactile sensations.

Auditory hallucinations, particularly the experience of hearing voices, are a common and often prominent feature of psychosis. Hallucinated voices may talk about, or to the person, and may involve several speakers with distinct personas. Auditory hallucinations tend to be particularly distressing when they are derogatory, commanding or preoccupying. However, the experience of hearing voices need not always be a negative one. Research has shown that the majority of people who hear voices are not in need of psychiatric help. The Hearing Voices Movement has subsequently been created to support voice hearers, regardless of whether they are considered to have a mental illness or not.

Delusions and Paranoia

Psychosis may involve delusional or paranoid beliefs. Karl Jaspers classified psychotic delusions into primary and secondary types. Primary delusions are defined as arising out of the blue and not being comprehensible in terms of normal mental processes, whereas secondary delusions may be understood as being influenced by the person's background or current situation (e.g., ethnic or sexual discrimination, religious beliefs, superstitious belief).

Thought disorder

Formal thought disorder describes an underlying disturbance to conscious thought and is classified largely by its effects on speech and writing. Affected persons may show pressure of speech (speaking incessantly and quickly), derailment or flight of ideas (switching topic mid-sentence or inappropriately), thought blocking, and rhyming or punning.

Lack of insight

One important and puzzling feature of psychosis is usually an accompanying lack of insight into the unusual, strange, or bizarre nature of the person's experience or behaviour. Even in the case of an acute psychosis, sufferers may be completely unaware that their vivid hallucinations and impossible delusions are in any way unrealistic. This is not an absolute, however; insight can vary between individuals and throughout the duration of the psychotic episode.

It was previously believed that lack of insight was related to general cognitive dysfunction or to avoidant coping style. Later studies have found no statistical relationship between insight and cognitive function, either in groups of people who only have schizophrenia, or in groups of psychotic people from various diagnostic categories.

In some cases, particularly with auditory and visual hallucinations, the patient has good insight, which makes the psychotic experience even more terrifying because the patient realizes that he or she should not be hearing voices, but is.

Schizophrenia is a serious illness for which the dominant feature, as perceived by the general public, is psychosis. It is schizophrenia that the average person thinks of in connection with terms such as "crazy" or "insane." The Web site for NAMI, the National Alliance for Mental Illness, at www.nami.org, describes schizophrenia as follows:

What is schizophrenia?

Schizophrenia is a medical illness that affects approximately 2.2 million American adults, or 1.1 percent of the population age 18 and older. Schizophrenia interferes with a person's ability to think clearly, to distinguish reality from fantasy, to manage emotions, make decisions, and relate to others. The first signs of schizophrenia typically emerge in the teenage years or early twenties. Most people with schizophrenia suffer chronically or episodically throughout their lives, and are often stigmatized by lack of public understanding about the disease. Schizophrenia is not caused by bad parenting or personal weakness. A person with schizophrenia does not have a "split personality," and almost all people with schizophrenia are not dangerous or violent towards others when they are receiving treatment. The World Health Organization has identified schizophrenia as one of the ten most debilitating diseases affecting human beings.

What are the symptoms of schizophrenia?

No one symptom positively identifies schizophrenia. All of the symptoms of this illness can also be found in other brain disorders. For example psychotic symptoms may be caused by the use of drugs, may be present in individuals with Alzheimer's Disease, or may be characteristics of a manic episode in bipolar disorder. However, when a doctor sees the symptoms of schizophrenia and carefully asseses the history and the course of the illness over six months, he or she can almost always make a correct diagnosis.

The symptoms of schizophrenia are generally divided into three categories, including positive, disorganized, and negative symptoms.[1]

- Positive Symptoms, or "psychotic" symptoms, include delusions and hallucinations because the patient has lost touch with reality in certain important ways. "Positive" as used here does not mean "good." Rather, it refers to having overt symptoms that should not be there. Delusions cause the patient to believe that people are reading their thoughts or plotting against them, that others are secretly monitoring and threatening them, or that they can control

---

[1]Whether this is in fact the best way to categorize the symptoms is a question around which debate remains. Some have argued that categorization into positive and negative symptoms is arbitrary, and introduces a type of bias that is more misleading than useful. That discussion, however, is beyond the scope of this book.

other people's minds. Hallucinations cause people to hear or see things that are not there.

- Disorganized Symptoms include confused thinking and speech, and behavior that does not make sense. For example, people with schizophrenia sometimes have trouble communicating in coherent sentences or carrying on conversations with others; move more slowly, repeat rhythmic gestures or make movements such as walking in circles or pacing; and have difficulty making sense of everyday sights, sounds and feelings.

- Negative Symptoms include emotional flatness or lack of expression, an inability to start and follow through with activities, speech that is brief and lacks content, and a lack of pleasure or interest in life. "Negative" does not, therefore, refer to a person's attitude, but to a lack of certain characteristics that should be there.

Schizophrenia is also associated with changes in cognition. These changes affect the ability to remember and to plan for achieving goals. Also, attention and motivation are diminished. The cognitive problems of schizophrenia may be important factors in long term outcome.

Schizophrenia also affects mood. Many individuals affected with schizophrenia become depressed, and some individuals also have apparent mood swings and even bipolar-like states. When mood instability is a major feature of the illness, it is called, schizoaffective disorder, meaning that elements of schizophrenia and mood disorders are prominently displayed by the same individual. It is not clear whether schizoaffective disorder is a distinct condition or simply a subtype of schizophrenia.

While the psychotic and cognitive problems attract the most attention, the negative symptoms of schizophrenia are truly crushing. The emotional flattening (blunted affect) and inability to feel pleasure (anhedonia) rob life of all value.

The treatment of schizophrenia and the treatment of psychosis are almost synonomous, and the medications prescribed for schizophrenia are known as *antipsychotic* medications, or *antipsychotics*. These same medications are often used to treat psychosis that arises from other conditions, most notably bipolar disorder. In fact, antipsychotic medications exert a mood-stabilizing effect that makes them effective for treating bipolar mania in general; however, their potential for serious side effects makes them generally less attractive than the standard mood stabilizers for this purpose.

Another, older term for antipsychotic that is often heard is neuroleptic, which means *calming*. *Neuroleptic* is less appropriate than *antipsychotic*, as other calming medications exist that work by different mechanisms than the antipsychotics. However, it is certainly the case that antipsychotic medications can be strongly tranquilizing. The tranquilizing effect varies widely between the different antipsychotics, and can be a benefit or drawback, depending on circumstances.

The challenge for treating schizophrenia lies in treating all categories of symptoms: psychosis, cognitive impairment, and negative symptoms, while at the same time avoiding undesirable side effects. The reality for people who have schizophrenia is that the ideal treatment usually does not happen, and they have to live with a compromise between benefits and drawbacks that is better than the untreated illness, but does not restore their quality of life to the norm.

This chapter will address treatments for schizophrenia and psychosis. The more general term of psychosis will be used with respect to the psychotic symptoms described above, and which may arise from disorders other than schizophrenia. The specific term of schizophrenia will be used only in connection with the illness of that name.

The two major categories of medications used to treat psychosis and schizophrenia are the *typical antipsychotics* and the *atypical antipsychotics*. The typical antipsychotics are older medications that have serious drawbacks, and are now seldom used for routine treatment of psychosis, although they are occasionally used for short-term treatment of anxiety or vomiting. The newer atypical antipsychotics are as effective at treating psychosis as the typical antipsychotics, while being less likely to have serious side effects. They also have the additional benefit of treating the negative symptoms of schizophrenia as well, restoring the capacity for emotion.

Because of their superior benefits and reduced drawbacks, the atypical antipsychotics are a major step forward in the treatment of schizophrenia and psychosis. However, they are still relatively dangerous drugs in comparison to medications used for other types of mental illness, such as depression, bipolar disorder, anxiety, and so forth. For this reason, they should be used with caution, and only when needed.

4.1 Causes of Schizophrenia and Psychosis

The causes of psychosis in general, and schizophrenia in particular, remain unknown. Psychotic symptoms can be induced temporarily by drugs, even in a healthy brain, so psychosis by itself probably can be explained in terms of abnormalities of brain chemistry. The illness of schizophrenia, however, is a permanent condition, and if the psychotic symtpoms manifest because of abnormalities in brain chemistry, then presumably the chemical abnormalities are themselves a manifestation of the illness. It seems likely, but has not been proven, that schizophrenia is ultimately a neurological problem, a set of symptoms resulting from damage or malformation of tissues in the brain, either congenital in nature, or caused by head injury or infection.

The following sections describe current theories about the neurochemistry of psychosis. Readers who are interested primarily in treatment, rather than causation, may wish to skip to the medication sections.

4.1.1 The Dopamine Hypothesis

The neurotransmitter dopamine plays the lead role in current theories regarding the neurochemical mechanisms responsible for psychosis. Many neurons in the brain send signals to adjacent neurons, from which they are separated by a synaptic gap, by emitting pulses of dopamine into the synaptic gap. Receptors on the receiving neuron are activated (register a signal) when dopamine molecules attach to them. While there are several dopamine receptors, the D_2 receptor is believed to play the most significant role in psychosis. (There are at least six dopamine receptors, currently labeled D_1, D_{2a}, D_{2b}, D_3, D_4, and D_5, of which D_3 and D_4 are subtypes of the more general category D_2.)

Primary evidence for the "dopamine hypothesis" for psychosis comes from the observation that all known effective antipsychotic medications are dopamine antagonists. More specifically, they block the D_2 dopamine receptor. (Each medication usually blocks other receptors, including dopamine receptors, as well, but the common theme among all antipsychotic medications is that all of them block the D_2 receptor.) For this reason, the primary chemical mechanism for treating psychosis is often referred to as "dopamine blockade." The effectiveness of antipsychotics in treating psychosis has led researchers to hypothesize that psychosis is at least partly a consequence of excess dopamine in certain parts of the brain.

The difficulty with treating psychosis, or schizophrenia, by stopping all dopamine-signal transmission (by blocking all dopamine receptors completely) is that it would "fix" the problem by removing the patient from the world of the living. Thus the difficulty faced by psychopharmacologists is to block enough of the undesirable dopamine signalling, while leaving the desirable signalling alone (or bolstering it, if not enough occurs). This is a tall order. The difficulty in achieving this goal is one reason that the current generation of antipsychotic medications, while helpful, is less than ideal in effectiveness. (Another reason is likely that psychosis, and certainly schizophrenia, involve more than the simplified picture of too much dopamine in some parts of the brain.)

4.1.2 The Four Dopamine Pathways

The brain, of course, is not a homogenous organ, but one that possesses a great deal of complexity. Different parts of the brain may respond quite differently to increases or decreases in neurotransmitter concentrations. This local variation in response is particularly important with regards to the treatment of psychosis and schizophrenia, which is tied to the function of four *dopamine pathways* in the brain.

A pathway is a bundle of nerve fibers that follow a particular path through the brain. The dopamine pathways are pathways for which dopamine-related signalling is especially important. As of this writing, four such dopamine pathways are known. The following sections describe the different dopamine pathways and their relationship to the symptoms of schizophrenia, as currently understood.

4.1.2.1 The Mesolimbic Dopamine Pathway

This pathway is believed to be involved in emotional disorders, delusions, thought disorders, and auditory hallucinations. Hyperactivity of the mesolimbic dopamine pathway is hypothesized to account for the positive symptoms of psychosis, and possibly hostility and excessive aggression as well. It is observed that reduction of dopamine-related signaling in this pathway by the blockade of D_2 receptors does lead to a decrease in the positive symptoms of psychosis.

4.1.2.2 The Mesocortical Dopamine Pathway

There is some evidence that some of the cognitive problems and negative symptoms of schizophrenia are due to an inadequate level of dopamine-related activity in this pathway. Assuming this is the case, it is not clear if the problem arises from low levels of dopamine, or damage to the neurons themselves (possibly due to poisoning from an excess of glutamate). If these hypotheses are correct, then increasing dopamine activity in this pathway could improve cognitive deficits and alleviate the negative symptoms.

4.1.2.3 The Nigrostriatal Dopamine Pathway

This pathway is part of the Extrapyramidal Nervous System. It controls motor movements. Dopamine deficiencies in this pathway produce movement problems (Extrapyramidal Symptoms, or EPS), such as Parkinson's disease. The types of movement problems caused by dopamine deficiencies include akinesia and bradykinesia (lack, or slowing, of movement, respectively), rigidity, tremor, akathisia (restlessness), and dystonia (twisting movements, especially of the face and neck).

Unfortunately, antipsychotic medications that blockade the D_2 receptor in this pathway can produce these movement disorders. If the D_2 blockade continues for an extended period of time, permanent dystonia (which continues even after the medication is stopped) can set in, a condition known as Tardive Dyskinesia.

It is believed that an excess of dopamine in this pathway causes hyperkinetic disorders, such as chorea, dyskinesias, and tics.

4.1.2.4 The Tuberoinfundibular Dopamine Pathway

Dopamine-related activity in this pathway inhibits prolactin release. Not surprisingly, pregnancy and childbirth lead to a reduction of dopamine activity in this pathway, thus increasing prolactin levels, and causing lactation, thus enabling breastfeeding. Undesirable dopamine reductions in this pathway (due to lesions or drugs) will also lead to prolactin increase (hyperprolactinemia), and can cause a variety of problems, such as galactorrhea (breast secretions), amenorrhea, and sexual dysfunction.

Conversely, increasing dopamine activity in this pathway acts to reduce prolactin levels, increase libido, and alleviate sexual dysfunction (see Chapter 5).

Once again, the undesirable consequences of dopamine suppression can occur as a result of antipsychotic medications that blockade dopamine in this area.

4.2   Treatments for Schizophrenia

The symptoms of schizophrenia (and psychosis) can only be alleviated by medical treatment. Therapy alone cannot address the underlying causes, which are neurological in origin. This is in contrast to the case of depression, as some instances of depression arise purely from factors within the capability of the individual to change, with help from a therapist. However, therapy does have a role to play in the overall management of schizophrenia. A good therapist can help a patient develop improved coping strategies for dealing with the illness. This is more important than it might sound, as the delusions and hallucinations severely distort the patient's capacity for judgment. A therapist's input can be of great value, as long as the patient is willing to work with the therapist, and take his input seriously. Unfortunately, the distortion of judgment characteristic of the psychotic experience (especially the anosognosia) may make it impossible for the patient to take the therapist seriously, or see him as other than a hostile and controlling influence.

The only technique, other than medication, that has been found to be effective in treating schizophrenia is that of electroconvulsive therapy, or ECT. This technique, which is described in Section 1.7.2, deserves careful consideration. Rightly or wrongly, ECT is often considered risky as a treatment for mental illness, but the medications used to treat schizophrenia are themselves considerably more dangerous than those used for, say, depression or bipolar disorder. The perceived risks of ECT may look more acceptable when compared to those of antipsychotic medications.

The experimental treatments described in Section 1.8 may be of interest as well, although they have not yet been demonstrated to be effective for schizophrenia.

The standard treatment for schizophrenia, and psychosis in general, is the use of antipsychotic medications, which are described in detail in the following sections.

Finally, one question that is seldom asked is whether schizophrenia *should* be treated. The question is not as simple it sounds, as the drawbacks of antipsychotic medications can be severe. Those with *mild* cases of shizophrenia, who are able to recognize and refuse to respond to (if not eliminate) illusory voices, may be better off developing coping strategies that allow them to function normally in the world, rather than taking antipsychotic medication. The patient and physician should consider the relative merits of medical treatment versus coping strategies, and make an educated decision as to which is most appropriate for the patient, instead of assuming that antipsychotic medication is always appropriate.

Similarly, those whose psychotic experiences are episodic, and who have the self-awareness to recognize when an episode is beginning, might choose to take (or increase their dose of) antipsychotic medication for the duration of the episode, instead of on a continuing basis.

4.3 The Dangers of Antipsychotic Medications

Compared to other categories of psychotropic medications, antipsychotic medications are the most dangerous. The possible dangers should not deter those who truly need antipsychotics from taking them, as the untreated illness is itself a very serious problem, but these medications should not be taken by those who have viable alternatives. The author is disturbed at the growing tendency to prescribe even the less dangerous atypical antipsychotics for the treatment of bipolar disorder and depression, when safer mood stabilizers and antidepressants are available.

While all psychotropic medications have undesirable side effects, even dangerous ones, the dangers of antipsychotics are uniquely troubling. The more noteworthy drawbacks are discussed below. The most serious threats to health (in terms of likelihood and severity) are Tardive Dyskinesia and Diabetes, both of which are incurable. Also of concern are the rarer possibilities of sudden death due to Neuroleptic Malignant Syndrome and QT Prolongation.

4.3.1 Tardive Dyskinesia

Tardive Dyskinesia (TD) is a disorder characterized by involuntary movements of the tongue, lips, face, upper body, and extremities.[2] Although the condition can occur naturally (albeit rarely), it most often occurs as a result of treatment with antipsychotic medications, and can arise from exposure to anticholinergic medications, toxins, illegal drugs, and other dangerous chemicals. Someone who has TD exhibits almost constant involuntary motions such as grimacing, smacking or pursing the lips, and protruding the tongue. Rapid movements of the eyelids (blinking), arms, legs, and upper body are also common, as are impairments to the movement of the hands and fingers. The condition is exceedingly distressing to the person who has it. Part of the distress comes from the condition itself, and part comes from the recoil of others who are appalled by the person's constant and involuntary writhing.

Exactly how antipsychotic medications cause TD is not known. It is clear that dopamine blockade is the ultimate cause, but how dopamine blockade leads to TD is not. Various mechanisms have been proposed, all of which involve modification of dopamine signalling mechanisms in the brain, or damage to brain tissue.

TD is treated by discontinuing or reducing the offending medication. The condition may persist for months or years after the medication is withdrawn, or even be permanent. Aside from medication change, the condition is incurable, and essentially untreatable. A variety of medications have produced ambiguous evidence

---

[2]*Dyskinesia* is the general term for abnormal movements, while *tardive* means *late*. The combination *tardive dyskinesia* means late-onset movement disorder, and refers to abnormal movements produced some time after antipsychotic medication has been taken.

for some symptomatic relief, including the atypical antipsychotic Clozapine, and benzodiazepines such as Clonazepam.

The extent to which people taking antipsychotic medications will develop TD is unclear, but substantial. There is some evidence to indicate that certain drugs (Haloperidol) are worse than others (Perphenazine), with the atypical antipsychotics being less likely to cause the condition than the typical antipsychotics. Aside from the variation among drugs, some estimates suggest that 15–30% of patients will develop TD on taking antipsychotics for three months or longer, while others suggest that each year of use increases the fraction of a treated population experiencing TD by 5%. The latter estimate in essence states that most people who use antipsychotics over the course of ten or more years will develop TD.

See www.emedicine.com and en.wikipedia.org/wiki/Tardive_dyskinesia for more details regarding Tardive Dyskinesia.

4.3.2 Diabetes

The atypical antipsychotics are thought to have lesser risks of some serious side effects, such as Tardive Dyskinesia or Neuroleptic Malignant Syndrome, and generally have fewer of the less dangerous side effects, as well as providing greater effectiveness at treating both the positive and negative symptoms of schizophrenia. So it comes as something of a surprise to find that they can cause diabetes, a condition *not* associated with the otherwise more dangerous typical antipsychotics.

The risk of diabetes appears significantly higher with the atypical antipsychotics, especially Clozapine and Olanzapine. One study indicated that 36% of patients treated with Clozapine developed diabetes over a five-year period.

As of this writing, evidence is ambiguous regarding the risk for Risperidone and Quetiapine. Ziprasidone and Aripiprazole are new enough that little information is available, but clinical trial data (pn.psychiatryonline.org/cgi/content/full/39/5/1-a) shows no evidence for diabetes risk at this time. It is likely that the risk varies among the atypical antipsychotics, but insufficient information is available to make an informed assessment at this time. Prudence suggests avoiding Clozapine and Olanzapine in favor of other atypical antipsychotics, and working with a physician to be alert for early warning signs of diabetes.

The mechanism by which these medications lead to diabetes is not known.

4.3.3 Neuroleptic Malignant Syndrome

Neuroleptic Malignant Syndrome (NMS) is a rare, but life threatening reaction to antipsychotic medication, consisting of fever, muscular rigidity, altered mental status, and dysfunction of the autonomic nervous system (see www.emedicine.com). It appears to be caused by blockade of the dopamine D_2 receptor in the hypothalamus, nigrostriatal pathway, and spinal cord, which leads to increased muscle rigidity, muscle-cell breakdown, muscle-tissue death and necrosis, tremor, elevated temperature, and dysfunction of the autonomic nervous system. This condition has only been observed in response to the use of antipsychotic medications. Atypical antipsychotics are less likely to produce this condition than the older typical antipsychotics, but the condition can occur with atypical antipsychotics.

The primary treatment of NMS is discontinuation of the antipsychotic medication, combined with supportive measures to alleviate the symptoms. The survival rate is at least 80%, and probably much higher. Unfortunately, resumption of antipsychotic medication is usually a necessity for the patient, in order to treat the original illness, but risks recurrence of NMS. The chance of recurrence can be decreased to below 30% by waiting more than two weeks before resuming the medication, and by switching to a different class of antipsychotic medication (one of the atypical antipsychotics).

Early warning signs that NMS may be developing include rigidity, fever, and changes of consciousness. The patient, family, and friends should be alert to any such signs, and report them to the patient's physician immediately.

4.3.4 QT Prolongation

QT Prolongation is an abnormal lengthening of the QT interval, which is the duration of the electrical activity that controls contraction of the heart muscle. This type of lengthening can occur due to an inherited medical condition (the Congenital Long QT syndrome) or in response to chemistry (medications, or abnormal levels of potassium, magnesium, and so forth). If the QT interval is prolonged too far beyond the norm, it can lead to a type of cardiac arrhythmia (heart malfunction) called Torsades de Pointes, a condition that can cause fainting or sudden death. (See the Arizona CERT Web site at www.arizonacert.org for details.)

Although many medications can cause some prolongation of the QT interval, the typical antipsychotic medications are among the worst offenders. Less is known about the risk of QT prolongation for the atypical antipsychotics, as they are of relatively recent origin, but they should be considered potentially dangerous, though probably less so than the typical antipsychotics.

The symptom of QT prolongation is heart palpitation, i.e., any obvious variation in rhythm or intensity of the heartbeat that is not due to normal causes, such as exercise or strong emotion. Anyone taking a medication known to cause serious QT prolongation should have an EKG test when experiencing an episode of heart palpitation. It is important to perform the EKG during the palpitation episode, which may require advance planning and coordination with your doctor, or even the use of portable heart monitors, if you tend to have short episodes. The EKG test can show whether the palpitations are due to QT prolongation or some other cause, and whether or not they are dangerous. If the EKG test does show significant QT prolongation, you may need to change medications.

4.4   Typical Antipsychotics

The *typical antipsychotics* are the first-generation treatments for schizophrenia and
psychosis. The first typical antipsychotic discovered, in the 1950s, was Chlorpromazine. Many other antipsychotic drugs with similar mechanisms, and with a variety of chemical structures, were discovered in the next few decades. They have
largely been replaced by the second-generation, *atypical antipsychotics*, for these
purposes, but remain useful for emergency sedation in cases of severe psychotic
episodes, and for uses unrelated to psychosis, such as treatment for severe vomiting,
pre-surgical anxiety, Tourette's Disorder, and even hiccups.

4.4.1   Mechanism

The typical antipsychotics work by blocking the dopamine D_2 receptors, a mechanism referred to as dopamine blockade. The blockade occurs throughout the brain,
affecting all four dopamine pathways. This indiscriminate blockade not only suppresses psychotic symptoms through its effects on the mesolimbic dopamine pathway
(Section 4.1.2.1), but also causes a variety of unpleasant symptoms due to blockading
the other dopamine pathways as well (Section 4.1.2).

4.4.2   Benefits

The primary purpose for which these medications were devised is to suppress psychotic symptoms, and they do this with reasonable effectiveness. Their waning use
as standard treatments for psychosis and schizophrenia has resulted in greater em-
phasis on their use in other areas, such as treatment for severe vomiting, pre-surgical
anxiety, Tourette's Disorder, and hiccups.

4.4.3   Principal Drawbacks

The drawbacks of chronic use of typical antipsychotics are many. The most serious
drawbacks are discussed in Section 4.3, namely Tardive Dyskinesia, Neuroleptic
Malignant Syndrome, and QT Prolongation.

Dopamine blockade also produces a variety of movement disorders, namely the
Extrapyramidal Symptoms (EPS). Tardive Dyskinesia is one particularly severe type
of EPS. Others include Parkinsonism, Dystonia, and Akathisia.

Parkinsonism is characterized by muscular rigidity, tremor, and impaired motor
control (i.e., difficulty grasping and manipulating objects, walking in a straight
line, and so forth).

Dystonia refers to any sustained and involuntary contraction of the muscles, which
leads to twisted and distorted posture.

Akathisia refers to motor restlessness, including quivering and an inability to sit still. In severe cases, akathisia makes resting and sleeping impossible.

EPS symptoms are often treated with beta blockers, benzodiazepines, and anticholinergic medications such as Benztropine, Trihexyphenidyl, and Diphenhydramine (a common, non-prescription allergy medicine, often sold under the name Benadryl).

The dopamine blockade also suppresses positive emotions, leading to anhedonia. (This is a particular and serious problem for people who have schizophrenia, as they are usually troubled by flattened affect to begin with.) Other effects include cognitive impairment (impaired capacity to think and concentrate). In fact, many of the side effects of typical antipsychotics are essentially the same as the negative symptoms of schizophrenia itself, which are exacerbated by the typical antipsychotics.

Other side effects are due to additional blockades, specifically of the muscarinic-cholinergic (M_1), Alpha 1 adrenergic (α_1), and histamine (H_1) receptors. These three mechanisms are also characteristic of the tricyclic antidepressants (TCAs), and are just as undesirable for antipsychotic medications.

The M_1 blockade can cause dry mouth, blurred vision, constipation, and cognitive impairment.

The Alpha 1 (α_1) blockade can cause orthostatic hypotension (low blood pressure on standing) and drowsiness.

The H_1 blockade can cause weight gain and drowsiness typical of antihistamine medications.

The undesirable side effects of typical antipsychotics are distressing at best, and crippling, dangerous, or even fatal at worst. The side effects are so serious that many patients have understandably chosen to skip the medication, and suffer the effects of psychosis as the lesser of two evils.

Danger! Chlorpromazine, Droperidol, Haloperidol, Mesoridazine, Pimozide, Thioridazine, and Zotepine have the highest risk level (of four) for causing QT Prolongation and serious abnormalities of heart rhythm. Medications at this risk level are believed to cause QT Prolongation. Medications with lower risk are preferred, and required for anyone who has Long QT Syndrome. If you cannot substitute a medication with lower risk, be alert for heart palpitations. If you experience palpitations, report them to your doctor immediately.

4.4.4   Medications

The largest family of typical antipsychotics is the Phenothiazine family.

Main Brand Name	Chemical Name	Chemical Type	Half Life	Wash-out Time	On-Label Uses	Off-Label Uses
Compazine	Prochlor-perazine	Pheno-thiazine	6 hours	2 days	Schizophrenia (psychosis); anxiety (non-psychotic); vomiting	
Mellaril	Thiori-dazine	Pheno-thiazine	23 hours	5 days	Schizophrenia (psychosis)	
Prolixin Injection	Fluphen-azine De-canoate	Pheno-thiazine	8 hours	40 days	Schizophrenia (psychosis)	
Serentil	Mesori-dazine	Pheno-thiazine	2 days	10 days	Schizophrenia (psychosis)	
Sparine	Promazine	Pheno-thiazine	6 hours	30 hours	Schizophrenia (psychosis)	
Stelazine	Trifluo-perazine	Pheno-thiazine	22 hours	5 days	Schizophrenia (psychosis); anxiety (non-psychotic)	
Thorazine	Chlor-promazine	Pheno-thiazine	30 hours	6 days	Schizophrenia (psychosis); vomiting; anxiety (pre-surgical); Por-phyria; Tetanus (adjunctive); Bipolar Dis-order (Manic phase); Hic-cups; explosive hyperexcitabil-ity in children; hyperactivity in children	anxiety (used as a sedative)
Trilafon	Perphen-azine	Pheno-thiazine	12 hours	3 days	Schizophrenia (psychosis); vomiting	

The second largest family of typical antipsychotics is the Thioxanthene family.

Main Brand Name	Chemical Name	Chemical Type	Half Life	Wash-out Time	On-Label Uses	Off-Label Uses
Depixol	Flupen-thixol	Thio-xanthene	35 hours	7 days	Schizophrenia (psychosis)	
Navane	Thiothixene	Thio-xanthene	30 hours	6 days	Schizophrenia (psychosis)	
Truxal	Chlorpro-thixene	Thio-xanthene	10 hours	2 days	Schizophrenia (psychosis); Bipolar Disorder (Manic phase)	

The remaining typical antipsychotics are all one-of-a-kind medications.

Main Brand Name	Chemical Name	Chemical Type	Half Life	Wash-out Time	On-Label Uses	Off-Label Uses
Haldol	Haloperidol	Butyro-phenone	21 hours	5 days	Schizophrenia (psychosis); Tourette's Disorder; explosive hyperexcitability in children; hyperactivity in children	
Haldol De-canoate	Haloperidol Decanoate	Butyro-phenone	3 weeks	15 weeks	Schizophrenia (psychosis)	
Loxitane	Loxapine	Dibenzoxa-zepine	4 hours	1 day	Schizophrenia (psychosis)	
Moban	Molindone	Dihydro-indolone	90 minutes	8 hours	Schizophrenia (psychosis)	

It is worth noting that some medications in the above chemical families, which have the standard antipsychotic mechanisms, are not approved by the Food and Drug Administration (FDA) for schizophrenia. They are used for conditions such as vomiting, anxiety, and Tourette's Disorder.

Medications approved for the control of severe vomiting, or prevention of vomiting in surgical procedures (anti-emetics), include the following:

Main Brand Name	Chemical Name	Chemical Type	Half Life	Wash-out Time	On-Label Uses	Off-Label Uses
Inapsine	Droperidol	Thio-xanthene	2 hours	10 hours	vomiting (in surgical and diagnostic procedures)	anxiety (used as a sedative)

Finally, Tourette's Disorder may be treated by the following:

Main Brand Name	Chemical Name	Chemical Type	Half Life	Wash-out Time	On-Label Uses	Off-Label Uses
Haldol	Haloperidol	Butyro-phenone	21 hours	5 days	Schizophrenia (psychosis); Tourette's Disorder; explosive hyperexcitability in children; hyperactivity in children	
Orap	Pimozide	Diphenyl-butyl-piperidine	55 hours	11 days	Tourette's Disorder	

4.4.5 Brand Names

Phenothiazine Antipsychotics

Chemical Name	Brand Names (Principal in Bold)
Chlor-promazine	**Thorazine**, Aminazin, Aminazine, Ampliactil, Chlordelazin, Chlorder-azin, Chlorpromados, Chlorpromanyl, Contomin, CPZ, Fenactil, Fenaktyl, Largactil, Novo-Chlorpromazine, Torazina
Fluphen-azine De-canoate	**Prolixin Injection**, Anatensol, Apo-Fluphenazine, Elinol, Fluorfenazine, Fluorophenazine, Fluorphenazine, Modecate, Moditen, Moditen Enanthate, Moditen Hcl, Omca, Pacinol, Permitil, Perphenazine, Pms Fluphenazine, Prolixin Decanoate, Prolixin Enanthate, Prolixine, Sevinol, Siqualine, Si-qualon, Tensofin, Triflumethazine, Valamina, Vespazine, Yespazine
Mesori-dazine	**Serentil**, Calodal, Lidanar, Lidanil, TPS-23, Thioridazien Thiomethyl Sul-foxide, Thioridazine Monosulfoxide Analog, Thioridazine Thiomethyl Sul-foxide, TPS23
Perphen-azine	**Trilafon**, Apo-Perphenazine, Apo Peram Tab, Chlorperphenazine, Decen-tan, Elavil Plus Tab, Emesinal, Etaperazin, Etaperazine, Ethaperazine, Etrafon, Etrafon-A, Etrafon-Forte, F-Mon, Fentazin, Fluphenazine, PZC, Perfenazina, Perfenazine, Perphenan, Perphenazin, Pms-Levazine, Pms Per-phenazine, Proavil, Thilatazin, Tranquisan, Triavil, Trifaron, Trilifan, Triph-enot
Prochlor-perazine	**Compazine**, Bayer A 173, Buccastem, Capazine, Chlormeprazine, Chlor-perazine, Combid, Compro, Emelent, Emetiral, Eskatrol, Kronocin, Me-terazin, Meterazin Maleate, Meterazine, Nipodal, Novamin, Pasotomin, Prochloroperazine, Prochlorpemazine, Prochlorperazin, Prochlorperazine edisylate, Prochlorperazine maleate, Prochlorpromazine, Procloperazine, Proclorperazine, Stemetil, Tementil, Temetid, Vertigon
Promazine	**Sparine**, AB, Ampazine, Berophen, Elmarin, Esmind, Esparin, Fraction, Liranol, Megaphen, Neo-Hibernex, Novomazina, Phenothiazine, Prazin, Prazine, Proma, Promactil, Promapar, Promazil, Promazin, Promaz-ina, Promwill, Propaphenin, Protactyl, Prozil, Psychozine, Romtiazin, Sanopron, Sinophenin, Sonazine, Tomil, Verophen, Vesprin, Wintermin
Thiori-dazine	**Mellaril**, Aldazine, Mallorol, Malloryl, Meleril, Mellaril-S, Mellarit, Mellerets, Mellerette, Melleretten, Melleril, Metlaril, Novoridazine, Orsanil, Ridazin, Ridazine, Sonapax, Stalleril, Thioridazin, Prolongatum, Thioridaz-inhydrochlorid, Thoridazine Hydrochloride, Tioridazin, Usaf Sz-3, Usaf Sz-B
Trifluo-perazine	**Stelazine**, Apo-Trifluoperazine, Eskazine, Eskazinyl, Fluoperazine, Ja-troneural, Modalina, Novo-Trifluzine, PMS Trifluoperazine, Stellazine, Synklor, Terfluzine, Trazine, Trifluoperazin, Trifluoperazina, Trifluo-romethylperazine, Trifluoroperazine, Trifluperazine, Triflurin, Trifluroper-izine, Triftazin, Triftazine, Triperazine, Triphtazin, Triphtazine, Triphtha-sine, Triphthazine, Tryptazine

Thioxanthene Antipsychotics

Chemical Name	Brand Names (Principal in Bold)
Chlorpro-thixene	**Truxal**, Alpha-Chlorprothixene, CPT, CPX, Chloroprothixene, Chlor-prothixen, Chlorprothixine, Chlorprotixen, Chlorprotixene, Chlorprotix-ine, Chlothixen, Cis-Chlorprothixene, Iaractan, Paxyl, Rentovet, Tactaran, Taractan, Tarasan, Tardan, Tranquilan, Traquilan, Trictal, Truxaletten, Truxil, Vetacalm
Flupen-thixol	**Depixol**, Depixol, Emergil, Fluanxol, Fluanxol Depot, Flupenthixole, Flu-pentixol, Flurentixol, Fluxanxol, Siplaril, Siplarol
Thio-thixene	**Navane**

Miscellaneous Antipsychotics

Chemical Name	Brand Names (Principal in Bold)
Halo-peridol	**Haldol**, ALDO, Aloperidin, Aloperidol, Aloperidolo, Aloperidon, Apo-Haloperidol, Bioperidolo, Brotopon, Dozic, Dozix, Einalon S, Eukystol, Ga-loperidol, Haldol Decanoate, Haldol La, Haldol Solutab, Halidol, Halojust, Halol, Halopal, Haloperido, Haloperidol Intensol, Halopidol, Halopoidol, Halosten, Keselan, Lealgin Compositum, Linton, Mixidol, Novo-Peridol, Pekuces, Peluces, Peridol, Pernox, Pms Haloperidol, Serenace, Serenase, Serenelfi, Sernas, Sernel, Sigaperidol, Ulcolind, Uliolind, Vesalium
Halo-peridol De-canoate	**Haldol Decanoate**
Loxapine	**Loxitane**, Cloxazepine, Dibenzacepin, Dibenzoazepine, Hydrofluoride 3170, Lossapina, Loxapac, Loxapin, Loxapina, Loxapine Succinate, Loxapinum, Loxepine, Loxitane C, Loxitane Im, Oxilapine
Molindone	**Moban**, Lidone

Anti-Emetics (for control of vomiting)

Chemical Name	Brand Names (Principal in Bold)
Droperidol	**Inapsine**, DHBP, Dehidrobenzperidol, Dehydrobenzperidol, Deidroben-zperidolo, Dihidrobenzperidol, Dridol, Droleptan, Halkan, Inappin, Inapsin, Innovan, Innovar, Innovar-Vet, Inopsin, Inoval, Leptanal, Leptofen, McN-JR 749, Properidol, Sintodril, Sintosian, Thalamonal, Thalamanol, Vetkalm

Tourette's Disorder Medication

Chemical Name	Brand Names (Principal in Bold)
Halo-peridol	**Haldol**, ALDO, Aloperidin, Aloperidol, Aloperidolo, Aloperidon, Apo-Haloperidol, Bioperidolo, Brotopon, Dozic, Dozix, Einalon S, Eukystol, Galoperidol, Haldol Decanoate, Haldol La, Haldol Solutab, Halidol, Halojust, Halol, Halopal, Haloperido, Haloperidol Intensol, Halopidol, Halopoidol, Halosten, Keselan, Lealgin Compositum, Linton, Mixidol, Novo-Peridol, Pekuces, Peluces, Peridol, Pernox, Pms Haloperidol, Serenace, Serenase, Serenelfi, Sernas, Sernel, Sigaperidol, Ulcolind, Uliolind, Vesalium
Pimozide	**Orap**, Haldol decanoate, Halomonth, Neoperidole, Opiran, Pimozidum, Primozida

4.5 Atypical Antipsychotics

The *atypical antipsychotics* are the second-generation treatments for psychosis and schizophrenia. The first atypical antipsychotic discovered, in the 1960s, was Clozapine, which received approval by the Food and Drug Administration (FDA) for use in treating schizophrenia in 1989. Several other atypical antipsychotics followed. Although the number of atypical antipsychotics available at this time is much smaller than the number of typical antipsychotics, these newer medications exhibit such improved effectiveness and decrease in undesirable side effects that they have largely replaced the older typical antipsychotics for the treatment of psychosis.

4.5.1 Mechanism

The standard mechanism for the atypical antipsychotics is a combination of serotonin and dopamine blockade; more specifically, blockade of both serotonin 2A and dopamine D_2 receptors. Many dopamine-producing neurons have serotonin 2A receptors. Their output of dopamine is regulated by signals from their serotonin receptors, with higher serotonin concentration leading to lower dopamine output. The serotonin blockade reduces the serotonin signal, and results in higher dopamine output, while the dopamine blockade suppresses dopamine signalling by blocking dopamine receptors. The two blockades are therefore at odds, simultaneously increasing dopamine concentration and decreasing dopamine effectiveness.

The odd opposition of effects plays out differently among the four dopamine pathways. The net effect, on average, is to reduce dopamine signalling in the mesolimbic dopamine pathway, increase dopamine signalling in the mesocortical and nigrostiratal dopamine pathways, and to fight roughly to a draw in the tuberoinfundibular dopamine pathway.

In more detail, the effects are as follows:

In the Mesolimbic Dopamine Pathway, the serotonin antagonism loses to the dopamine antagonism. The dopamine D_2 blockade successfully suppresses positive psychotic symptoms, just as the typical antipsychotics do.

In the Mesocortical Dopamine Pathway, the serotonin antagonism wins quite strongly over the dopamine antagonism, causing a net increase in dopamine activity. Not only does the increase in dopamine activity prevent undesirable side effects of dopamine blockade, but can actually improve the negative symptoms of psychosis, restoring the lost capacity for emotion and pleasure.

In the Nigrostriatal Dopamine Pathway, the serotonin antagonism wins over the dopamine antagonism, increasing the amount of dopamine available (relative to what a typical antipsychotic would do), and thus reducing the danger or severity of Extrapyramidal symptoms (including tardive dyskinesia).

In the Tuberoinfundibular Dopamine Pathway, the effects of the simultaneous serotonin and dopamine blockade on prolactin release are mixed. The dopamine blockade acts to increase prolactin, while the serotonin blockade acts, separately, to decrease prolactin. The net effect is that prolactin release is reduced relative to the typical antipsychotics. Compared to the case where no antipsychotic medication is used, the atypical antipsychotics may or may not reduce prolactin emission. The net effect on libido may be positive, negative, or insignificant.

The antipsychotic medication Amisulpride is an exception to the above pattern. It has the reduced side-effect profile of the atpyical antipsychotics, and is therefore categorized with them in terms of its effectiveness, but its mechanism is different. Amisulpride blockades the post-synaptic dopamine D_2 receptor, as do the other atypical antipsychotics, but has no effect on serotonin receptors. At the same time, it blockades D_2 and D_3 pre-synaptic receptors that also regulate dopamine production, causing an increase in dopamine production. Thus Amisulpride demonstrates an alternate approach to the combination of dopamine D_2 blockade and increased dopamine emission, relative to the other atypical antipsychotic medications.

Paliperodine is also the major active metabolite of risperidone, another antipsychotic medication, and thus its effects should be very similar to those of risperidone.

4.5.2   Benefits

These medications suppress psychotic symptoms with reasonable effectiveness. Unlike the typical antipsychotics, the atypical antipsychotics can alleviate the negative symptoms of schizophrenia as well, improving, rather than suppressing, the capacities to think and feel emotion, which is a tremendous benefit. Also unlike the typical antipsychotics, the atypical antipsychotics have less propensity to cause Neuroleptic Malignant Syndrome and extrapyramidal symptoms (movement disorders), including Tardive Dyskinesia.

Paliperodine may have fewer side effects than risperidone, but evidence is too limited to make a definitive statement.

4.5.3   Principal Drawbacks

Unfortunately, the atypical antipsychotics can cause diabetes, something not observed with the older typical antipsychotics (see Section 4.3.2). Also, while the atypical antipsychotics are less likely to exhibit the undesirable side effects of the older typical antipsychotics, *less likely* does not mean *never*. Thus all of the drawbacks of the typical antipsychotics described in Section 4.4.3 remain for the atypical antipsychotics as well, but with generally lesser frequency and severity.

It is safe to say that the atypical antipsychotics represent a major step forward in the treatment of psychosis and schizophrenia, but still fall well short of the ideal.

Warning! Clozapine, Quetiapine, Risperidone, and Ziprasidone have the second-highest risk level (of four) for causing QT Prolongation and serious abnormalities of heart rhythm. Medications at this risk level have been associated with QT Prolongation, but not proven to cause it. The risk for QT Prolongation is not considered high, but medications with lower risk are preferred, especially for anyone who has Long QT Syndrome. If you cannot substitute a medication with lower risk, be alert for heart palpitations. If you experience palpitations, report them to your doctor immediately.

4.5.4 Medications

Main Brand Name	Chemical Name	Chemical Type	Half Life	Wash-out Time	On-Label Uses	Off-Label Uses
Abilify	Aripiprazole	Benzi-soxazole	4 days	20 days	Schizophrenia (psychosis)	
Clozaril	Clozapine		12 hours	3 days	Schizophrenia (psychosis), treatment-resistant; suicidal behavior	
Dolmatil	Sulpiride	Benzamide	8 hours	2 days	Schizophrenia (psychosis)	
Geodon	Ziprasidone	Benzi-soxazole	7 hours	35 hours	Schizophrenia (psychosis); Bipolar Disorder (Manic phase); agitation in schizophrenic patients	
Invega	Paliper-idone	Benzi-soxazole	1 day	5 days	Schizophrenia (psychosis)	
Risperdal	Risperidone	Benzi-soxazole	20 hours	4 days	Schizophrenia (psychosis); Bipolar Disorder (Manic phase)	Asperger's Syndrome; Autism; Depression (psychotic)
Serdolect	Sertindole		3 days	15 days	Schizophrenia (psychosis)	
Seroquel	Quetiapine	Benzi-soxazole	6 hours	30 hours	Schizophrenia (psychosis); Bipolar Disorder (Manic and Depressive phases)	
Solian	Amisulpride	Benzamide	12 hours	3 days	Schizophrenia (psychosis)	
Zoleptil	Zotepine	Dibenzo-thiepine	15 hours	3 days	None (Investigational)	Schizophrenia (psychosis)
Zyprexa	Olanzapine		30 hours	6 days	Schizophrenia (psychosis); Bipolar Disorder (Manic phase)	Obsessive-Compulsive Disorder; Autism (for behavioral disorders)

4.5.5 Brand Names

Chemical Name	Brand Names (Principal in Bold)
Amisul-pride	**Solian**
Aripip-razole	**Abilify**, Abilitat, OPC 31
Clozapine	**Clozaril**, Asaleptin, Clozapin, Fazaclo ODT, Iprox, Leponex, Lepotex
Olanza-pine	**Zyprexa**, Olansek, Symbyax, Zydis, Zyprexa Intramuscular, Zyprexa Zydis
Paliper-idone	**Invega**
Quetiapine	**Seroquel**, Quetiapin hemifumarate, Quetiapine fumarate, Quetiapine hemi-fumarate
Risper-idone	**Risperdal**, Risperdal Consta, Risperdal M-Tab, Risperidal M-Tab, Risperi-dona, Risperidonum, Risperin, Rispolept, Rispolin, Sequinan
Sertindole	**Serdolect**
Sulpiride	**Dolmatil**, Abilit, Aiglonyl, Alimoral, Calmoflorine, Championyl, Coolspan, Darleton, Desmenat, Dobren, Dogmatil, Dogmatyl, Dresent, Eclorion, Eglonil, Eglonyl, Enimon, Equilid, Eusulpid, Fardalan, Fidelan, Guastil, Isnamide, Kylistro, Levobren, Levopraid, Levosulpirida, Levosulpiride, Levosulpiridum, Lisopiride, Mariastel, Meresa, Miradol, Mirbanil, Misulvan, Neogama, Norestran, Normum, Nufarol, Omiryl, Omperan, Ozoderpin, Psicocen, Pyrikappl, Pyrkappl, Restful, Sernevin, Splotin, Stamonevrol, Sulpirid, Sulpirida, Sulpiridum, Sulpitil, Sulpride, Sulpyrid, Suprium, Sursumid, Synedil, Trilan, Valirem, Zemorcon
Ziprasi-done	**Geodon**, Zeldox
Zotepine	**Zoleptil**

Chapter 5

Sexual Dysfunction

The reader may wonder why a book on psychotropic medications has a chapter on sexual dysfunction. There are two reasons:

- Many of the psychotropic medications discussed elsewhere in this book (especially antidepressants and antipsychotics) cause serious sexual problems, so alleviation of those problems is clearly an appropriate topic.

- Many of the medications that are useful for treating sexual disorders are themselves psychotropic medications, although they are primarily prescribed for other problems.

Broadly speaking, the term "sexual dysfunction" refers to any problem or condition that prevents a satisfactory sex life. It includes any problem, physical or emotional, that prevents an individual or couple from enjoying sexual activity. Since every person is likely to experience transient sexual difficulties on occasion, a sexual problem is considered to be a sexual dysfunction *disorder* only if it is sustained over time.

Wikipedia (en.wikipedia.org/wiki/Sexual_dysfunction) has the following to say about the different categories of sexual dysfunction.

Sexual dysfunction disorders are generally classified into four categories: sexual desire disorders, sexual arousal disorders, orgasm disorders, and sexual pain disorders.

1. **Sexual desire disorders** or decreased libido can be caused by a decrease in normal estrogen (in women) or testosterone (in both men and women) production. Other causes may be aging, fatigue, pregnancy, medications (such as the SSRIs) or psychiatric conditions, such as depression and anxiety.

2. **Sexual arousal disorders** were previously known as frigidity in women and impotence in men, though these have now been replaced

with less judgmental terms. Impotence is now known as erectile dysfunction, and frigidity has been replaced with a number of terms describing specific problems with, for example, desire or arousal.

For both men and women, these conditions can manifest as an aversion to, and avoidance of, sexual contact with a partner. In men, there may be partial or complete failure to attain or maintain an erection, or a lack of sexual excitement and pleasure in sexual activity.

There may be medical causes to these disorders, such as decreased blood flow or lack of vaginal lubrication. Chronic disease can also contribute, as well as the nature of the relationship between the partners. As the success of sildenafil (Viagra) attests, most erectile disorders in men are primarily physical, not psychological conditions.

3. **Orgasm disorders** are a persistent delay or absence of orgasm following a normal sexual excitement phase. The disorder can occur in both women and men. Again, the SSRI antidepressants are frequent culprits – these can delay the achievement of orgasm or eliminate it entirely.

4. **Sexual pain disorders** affect women almost exclusively and are known as dyspareunia (painful intercourse) and vaginismus (an involuntary spasm of the muscles of the vaginal wall that interferes with intercourse). Dyspareunia may be caused by insufficient lubrication (vaginal dryness) in women.

This chapter addresses the use of prescription medications that may be used to treat some sexual problems. It is not a comprehensive guide to the treatment of sexual dysfunction; in particular, it does not address psychological problems, or sexual pain disorders, for which the reader is advised to look elsewhere. This chapter focuses more narrowly on medical treatment for sexual desire disorder (low libido, also known as Hypoactive Sexual Desire), sexual arousal disorder (such as Erectile Dysfunction, or ED), and orgasm disorder (i.e., Anorgasmia, or difficulty achieving orgasm).

While the primary motivation for this chapter is to address sexual dysfunction caused by psychotropic medications (primarily antidepressants), many of the treatments described are also of value to those whose sexual problems do not arise from medication.

5.1 Solutions for Sexual Dysfunction in General

The solutions described in this section are appropriate for sexual dysfunction in general, meaning whether or not the dysfunction arises from antidepressant medication.

While these medications can normally be taken in conjunction with an antidepressant, individual exceptions may occur, and it is important to discuss possible drug interactions with your physician.

5.1.1 Treating Sexual Arousal Disorders

Arousal disorders are most obvious in men, where they take the form of Erectile Dysfunction (ED). ED refers to the inability to develop and sustain an erection, and by definition, refers to men only. Medications that treat ED are available, and the degree to which they work is obvious to the men who take them. These medications have brought great benefit to men who have normal sexual desires, but suffer from ED.

The following sections refer explicitly to ED, rather than arousal disorders in general, because they reflect the language of the prescribing literature for the medications. However, women also experience arousal disorders, although the symptoms are less obvious than those of ED.

Women may experience arousal disorders in the form of dryness or insufficient engorgement, which cause discomfort, and understandable reluctance to engage in sexual activity. Fortunately, the medications (vasodilators) that are useful for ED in men can improve vaginal engorgement and lubrication for women.

Arousal desires in men and women are primarily physical in nature. Psychological problems can certainly lead to arousal problems, but in such cases, the psychological problems are not themselves arousal problems, and must be treated differently.

It is important to realize that medications for arousal disorders are not "aphrodisiacs." They do not help problems of low libido, unlike some other medications described in this chapter.

5.1.1.1 PDE5 Inhibitors

The big breakthrough in the treatment of ED was the discovery of vasodilators that increase blood flow to the penis. These vasodilators increase the concentration of cyclic guanosine monophosphate (cGMP), a chemical that relaxes the smooth muscles, and increases blood flow to the penis following sexual stimulation. They work by selectively inhibiting a chemical named phosphodiesterase type 5 (PDE5), which destroys cGMP.

The PDE5 inhibitors are very effective medications, with a high success rate. They differ primarily in terms of how quickly their effects are noticed, and how long they last. In all cases, benefits typically are observed in less than an hour. Standard dosing instructions are to take the medication an hour before sexual activity. The benefits may last from a few hours to over a day, depending on the medication and individual variation in response. In general, the longer the half life, the longer the benefits are likely to last.

The most commonly noted side effects are headache and flushing. These effects are rarely serious enough to impair sexual function (or be a health hazard). Excessively prolonged erections (priapism) are unlikely but a possibility, and immediate medical treatment should be sought if erection persists for more than an hour after sexual activity. Prolonged states of erection (lasting more than an hour) can cause serious and irreversible damage to the penis, and are a medical emergency that require immediate treatment.

Warning! Vardenafil has the second-highest risk level (of four) for causing QT Prolongation and serious abnormalities of heart rhythm. Medications at this risk level have been associated with QT Prolongation, but not proven to cause it. The risk for QT Prolongation is not considered high, but medications with lower risk are preferred, especially for anyone who has Long QT Syndrome. If you cannot substitute a medication with lower risk, be alert for heart palpitations. If you experience palpitations, report them to your doctor immediately.

Main Brand Name	Chemical Name	Chemical Type	Half Life	Wash-out Time	On-Label Uses	Off-Label Uses
Cialis	Tadalafil		18 hours	4 days	Erectile Dysfunction	
Levitra	Vardenafil		5 hours	1 day	Erectile Dysfunction	
Viagra	Sildenafil		8 hours	2 days	Erectile Dysfunction	

5.1.1.2   PGE1 Vasodilators

Another type of vasodilator that is useful for treating ED is the chemical prostaglandin E1 (PGE1), which occurs naturally in the body. An increase in PGE1 concentration in the penis relaxes the smooth muscles, and increases blood flow to the penis following sexual stimulation.

When used to treat ED, PGE1 is supplied in the form of a very small urethral suppository. The half-life is very short, so the medication should be used immediately before sexual activity. Benefits are observed in 5–10 minutes, and last for 30–60 minutes.

The most common side effect is pain in the penis, urethra, or testicles, which is usually mild and temporary.

Main Brand Name	Chemical Name	Chemical Type	Half Life	Wash-out Time	On-Label Uses	Off-Label Uses
Muse	Alprostadil		5 minutes	25 minutes	Erectile Dysfunction	

5.1.1.3 Apomorphine

Apomorphine is a dopamine agonist used to treat Parkinson's disease (as Apokyn, an injectable medication) and ED (as Uprima, in sub-lingual tablet form). Unlike vasodilators, Apomorphine stimulates dopamine receptors in the brain. Thus Apomorphine can provide a boost in libido which, in turn, promotes erection. Apomorphine may be useful in situations where vasodilators are not, and vice versa.

Apomorphine is administered by sub-lingual table or injection. The half-life is short, so it should be taken thirty minutes before sexual activity. Benefits are normally observed within 10–20 minutes, and may last for a few hours.

The most common side effect of Apomorphine is nausea.

Main Brand Name	Chemical Name	Chemical Type	Half Life	Wash-out Time	On-Label Uses	Off-Label Uses
Uprima	Apomorphine		40 minutes	4 hours	Parkinson's Disease	Erectile Dysfunction

Although Apomorphine may be useful for ED, it is not clear that it is more effective for this purpose than other dopamine agonists. The sub-lingual administration and rapid onset of effect are convenient when compared to the vasodilators, but the short half life means that the benefits are not sustained. This may not seem like a problem relative to the vasodilators, but other dopamine agonists have much longer half lives, and may provide the same benefits as Apomorphine on a sustained, rather than intermittent, basis.

The reason Apomorphine is listed separately here, rather than being grouped with the other dopamine agonists, is because the Uprima formulation has been developed specifically for the treatment of Erectile Dysfunction, and because it is too short-lived to be of much use for the treatment of depression. However, it is entirely possible that dopamine agonists with longer half-lives will prove more beneficial for both ED and libido problems. (See Section 5.1.2.2.)

5.1.1.4 Yohimbine

Yohimbine is a prescription medication derived from the Yohimbe tree. It is an α-adrenergic antagonist, meaning it blocks α (alpha) norepinephrine receptors. Yohimbine also has monoamine-oxidase inhibitory effects, and may cause a dangerous increase in blood pressure in conjunction with other medications, or foods that contain tyramine (see www.inchem.org/documents/pims/pharm/yohimbin.htm, or Section 2.4.4.2, for details).

Yohimbine has multiple effects on the body. It is a stimulant, and increases heart rate and blood pressure. Like all stimulants, Yohimbine may increase anxiety.

Yohimbine is not a vasodilator, but has similar benefits to the vasodilators for ED: it increases blood flow to the penis, and promotes erection. The rapid absorption (about 10 minutes) and short half-life means that Yohimbine should be taken immediately before sexual activity.

The most common side effects of Yohimbine are nausea, shakiness, tension, and anxiety. Overdoses can produce unconsciousness, dizziness, confusion. Excessively prolonged erections (priapism) are unlikely but a possibility, and immediate medical treatment should be sought if erection persists for more than an hour after sexual activity. Prolonged states of erection (lasting more than an hour) can cause serious and irreversible damage to the penis, and are a medical emergency that require immediate treatment.

Given Yohimbine's complex behavior, it is not a first choice for the treatment of ED, but may be useful if other medications prove ineffective.

Main Brand Name	Chemical Name	Chemical Type	Half Life	Wash-out Time	On-Label Uses	Off-Label Uses
Yocon	Yohimbine		45 minutes	4 hours	Erectile Dysfunction	

5.1.2 Treating Sexual Desire Disorders

The condition of low or absent sexual desire has been given many names, such as low libido, or *Inadequate Sexual Desire* (ISD). The term that will be used here is *Hypoactive Sexual Desire* (HSD). Whatever the name, it is important to realize that the level of sexual desire varies widely. The definition of healthy sexual desire, and therefore of inadequate sexual desire, depends on the satisfaction of the person or couple involved. An individual's level of desire is only "low" if it makes the individual, or couple, unhappy.

HSD often arises from psychological problems, such as marital problems, past trauma, or other life experiences; however, psychological treatments for HSD are beyond the scope of this book.

A number of medications are useful for treating HSD that arises from physical, rather than psychological, problems, although none of them have been not approved specifically by the Food and Drug Administration (FDA) for this purpose. (All of the medications described below have been officially approved by the FDA for other purposes.) However, physicians frequently use their own judgment and prescribe medications for off-label uses, so there is nothing unusual about the practice.

Antidepressant medications that increase serotonin concentration (serotonergic antidepressants) frequently cause HSD. Some of the medications described below help primarily with HSD that is due to serotonergic antidepressants; some are useful whether or not such antidepressants are the cause; and some are useful only for people who are not taking these antidepressants.

5.1.2.1 Hormone Therapy

Many endocrine (hormonal) disorders have the potential to cause HSD. If HSD is not an obvious consequence of life circumstances, medication, or illness, then an endocrine disorder is a likely culprit. Thus the first step in the medical treatment of HSD is to see a doctor for a thorough examination, to determine if the problem is hormonal in nature. If at all possible, it is better to see an Endocrinologist than a General Practitioner, as the latter generally lack the knowledge to diagnose the more complex hormonal problems.

Common endocrine problems that can cause HSD include thyroid disorders of various kinds, low testosterone levels, and high prolactin levels. These and other endocrine problems can be treated successfully by a competent Endocrinologist. (However, HSD that arises from serotonergic antidepressants is not treatable by hormone therapy.)

One should look for other medical treatments for HSD only if endocrine problems have been ruled out. The following sections assume either that HSD has no endocrine component, or that any endocrine problems that exist have been treated, but the HSD remains unresolved.

5.1.2.2 Dopaminergic Medications

The hormone prolactin serves useful purposes in the body, most notably in stimulating milk production in pregnant and nursing women. However, an excess of prolactin can sharply decrease libido in both men and women. Since the rate at which prolactin is produced decreases as dopamine concentration increases, one effective way to treat HSD is by the use of dopaminergic medications. These medications either increase dopamine concentration, or (in the case of dopamine agonists) provide a substitute for dopamine. Dopaminergic medications are perhaps the best approximations to the concept of aphrodisiacs as any prescription medications available today.

The dopaminergic medications described in this section may be useful for HSD problems whether or not the problems are caused by serotonergic antidepressants. They can usually be taken in conjunction with antidepressant medications.

The medication Levodopa, or l-dopa, is not included in the list of useful dopaminergic medications. The omission may seem odd, given that l-dopa is a dopamine precursor, which is converted to dopamine. Like the dopamine agonists and Selegiline, it is used to treat Parkinson's disease. The reason it is not suggested for the treatment of sexual dysfunction is because there has been some speculation that l-dopa may cause degradation of dopamine-emitting neurons over time. Its use in Parkinson's disease may be required, but its use for other purposes is not advised.

5.1.2.2.1 Bupropion (Wellbutrin) This antidepressant (see Section 2.5.7) provides a modest increase in dopamine concentration. It is the least effective of the dopaminergic augmentations discussed in this section, but because it is a standard antidepressant, it is also the most widely-used, and familiar to physicians.

5.1.2.2.2 Dopamine Agonists These medications act as substitutes for dopamine, rather than increase its concentration (see Section 2.7). Like Selegiline (Sections 2.4.3 and 5.1.2.2.3), they can have a dramatic effect on libido; unlike Selegiline, they may be used freely with SSRIs or other serotonergic medications. Also unlike Selegiline, they do not increase norepinephrine levels, and thus have no effect on energy or concentration.

As noted in Section 2.7, Amantadine is the weakest of the dopamine agonists, while the others may be expected to be of comparable effectiveness. Of the latter, Cabergoline is considered to be the most easily tolerated (least likely to cause unpleasant side effects).

5.1.2.2.3 Selegiline Selegiline, a selective MAO inhibitor (Section 2.4.3), is another dopaminergic medication. While it has been known since 1965, and long used to treat Parkinson's disease, it has only recently been approved by the Food and Drug Administration (FDA) for the treatment of depression, and only in transdermal form (i.e., supplied by the Emsam skin patch). However, the oral form provides comparable benefits, and is readily available. The two forms should be equally effective in treating HSD.

Selegiline is noteworthy as the only prescription medication that dramatically increases the concentration of dopamine in the brain (aside from l-dopa), without affecting serotonin (except at high doses). As a result, it can have a dramatic effect on libido. It is also a stimulating medication, meaning that it improves energy and concentration, because it also increases the concentration of norepinephrine. Like the dopamine agonists of Sections 2.7 and 5.1.2.2, Selegiline is about as close to the concept of an aphrodisiac as any prescription medication currently available.

Unfortunately, standard prescribing requirements state that Selegiline cannot be used in conjunction with any other antidepressant (although one could make the argument that this proscription probably should apply, at least at lower doses, only to serotonergic antidepressants). The reason for this prohibition is that it is in the category of MAO inhibitors, and MAO inhibitors are notorious for their drug-interaction problems. On the other hand, while it is certainly true that the more well-known MAOIs (Isocarboxazid, Phenelzine, and Tranylcypromine) must not be taken with, say, an SSRI, as the combination can cause an overdose of serotonin known as Serotonin Syndrome, it is also the case that Selegiline does not affect serotonin levels significantly at low doses (10 mg or less). Thus it seems plausible that one might be able to take Selegiline along with an SSRI. However, this combination is currently forbidden in standard medical practice, and must be regarded as such pending further investigation.

5.1.2.3 Partial Serotonin Agonists

Buspirone (BuSpar) has been found to be useful for problems of both HSD and Anorgasmia, whether or not the problems are caused by serotonergic antidepressants. It can usually be taken in conjunction with antidepressant medications.

Buspirone acts as an agonist to serotonin 1A receptors, and an antagonist to α norepinephrine receptors. Exactly why Buspirone alleviates sexual dysfunction is not clear, but it has been found to be beneficial.

Main Brand Name	Chemical Name	Chemical Type	Half Life	Wash-out Time	On-Label Uses	Off-Label Uses
BuSpar	Buspirone		24 hours	5 days	anxiety	Sexual Dysfunction

5.2 Antidepressant-Induced Sexual Dysfunction

As Section 1.4.1 indicated, medications that increase the concentration of serotonin frequently have adverse effects on sexuality. The sexual problems that can occur include loss of libido (Hypoactive Sexual Desire), erectile dysfunction, and anorgasmia. A particular person may experience any or all of these effects, to any degree.

Psychiatrists and pharmaceutical companies were slow to recognize (or admit) that medications used to treat depression could cause sexual problems. As of this writing, the problems are now well known, and are clearly a consequence of the increase in serotonin concentration, which has the following effects:

- The increased concentration of serotonin stimulates the serotonin 2A (5-HT2A) receptors in the brain. Stimulation of these receptors in neurons that produce dopamine causes them to decrease the rate at which they produce it, resulting in lower dopamine concentration.

  Dopamine plays a major role in the experience of pleasure, and of sexual desire in particular. The reduction in dopamine (most notably, in the Tuberoinfundibular Dopamine Pathway) leads to an increase in prolactin concentration, which reduces libido. The dopamine decrease can also impair the ability to feel pleasure in general, a condition known as anhedonia.

- The increase in serotonin concentration throughout the body stimulates serotonin receptors in the spinal cord, which inhibits orgasm and ejaculation.

Unfortunately, there is no consensus on how to alleviate sexual dysfunction induced by psychotropic medications. As of this writing, too little research has been done on treatment strategies for well-tested methods to emerge.

However, the situation is not quite as bleak as it may seem. Although their effectiveness may not always have been confirmed by clinical studies, solutions for overcoming sexual dysfunction do exist. They aren't perfect, and none of them is guaranteed to work for everyone, but there is substantial anecdotal evidence that each works for some people. Many such solutions are described in this chapter.

5.3 Solutions for Dysfunction Caused by Antidepressants

The question naturally arises as to which solution is likely to be the most effective. Unfortunately, the current state of medical science does not provide much guidance in this area. Common sense suggests the following rough guidelines:

- Lack of sexual desire; i.e., Hypoactive Sexual Desire (HSD): The medications described in Section 5.1.2 may suffice to resolve the problem, when taken in conjunction with the antidepressant. This is a common *augmentation* strategy. If this approach does not work, then one of the solutions described below may help.

- Other types of sexual dysfunction; i.e., Anorgasmia and Erectile Dysfunction (ED): These problems are unlikely to respond to the medications of Section 5.1.2, and will require one of the solutions described below.

Note that it is important to discuss any approach with your doctor before trying it, especially when issues of drug interactions arise. Your doctor should know whether a particular solution is safe for you.

The solutions described in this section are appropriate only for cases where sexual dysfunction is caused by an antidepressant that increases serotonin concentration. Most should be tried only after enough time has passed (four to six weeks) to discover whether the dysfunction is a temporary problem associated with starting the medication, or a permanent side effect of the medication. A particular solution may help with none, some, or all of the types of sexual dysfunction, depending on the individual's response. In addition, the medications described in Section 5.1 may also be used, unless otherwise indicated.

See also www.sexualwholeness.com/isw/resources/7092/boyarsky2000.pdf for a good description of these treatment strategies.

5.3.1 Dose Time Change

Changing the time of day at which the medication is taken may help, if the medication has a short enough half-life. (For example, Fluvoxamine, i.e. Luvox, has a half-life of 16 hours.) Taking the day's dose just after the usual time for sexual activity (for example, at bedtime) guarantees that the amount of the medication in the body, and any consequent sexual impairment, is at its lowest level at that time.

This approach will not work for medications with half-lives that are much longer than the standard daily dosing interval, such as Fluoxetine (Prozac). (On the other hand, Fluoxetine may also be taken on a weekly basis, an approach that might provide a longer window of sexual capability towards the end of each week.)

5.3.2 Drug Holidays

This approach is also most appropriate for medications with shorter half-lives. Omitting the daily dose for one or two days every week may allow for more normal sexual function during those days.

Drug holidays have some drawbacks. First, it increases the likelihood that depression may return during the "holiday" periods. Second, it may interfere with the treatment of depression in general. Third, some medications may produce unpleasant withdrawal effects during this period, which eliminate or outweigh any possible benefits. For these reasons, it is important to work closely with your doctor when attempting this approach.

5.3.3 Dose Reduction

One of the most obvious techniques for improving sexual function is to reduce the dose of the medication that is causing the problem. It may be, for example, that sexual dysfunction becomes a problem at a 30 mg dose, while a 20 mg dose suffices to treat the illness. In this case, reducing the dosage to the minimum required to achieve the benefits may result in escaping the sexual problem.

5.3.4 Medication Change

Another obvious technique for treating sexual dysfunction produced by a medication is to try a different medication. Assuming that the medication is a serotonergic antidepressant, there are a few possible cases, ordered by decreasing likelihood of improvement in sexual function.

1. Switch to a non-serotonergic antidepressant, such as Bupropion (Section 2.5.7), Selegiline (Section 5.1.2.2.3), or Tianeptine (Section 2.5.9). This approach is likely to work very well, as far as sexual function is concerned, but if the particular case of depression requires a serotonergic medication for successful treatment, then this approach is not an option. (Note, however, that Selegiline does increase serotonin concentration when taken at sufficiently high doses, so this is a possible option for people who do require a serotonin boost.)

2. Switch to, or add, Mirtazapine (Section 2.5.8), Nefazodone (Section 2.5.4), or Trazodone (Section 2.5.4). (These tricyclic antidepressants (and, to a lesser extent, Nortriptyline) blockade the serotonin 5-HT2A receptors specifically. As a result, they provide serotonergic benefits that alleviate depression, but

with less impact on sexual function. Since SSRI-induced insomnia is also associated with stimulation of the 5-HT2A receptors, these medications can alleviate the insomnia as well.)

Drawbacks of Mirtazapine include the possibility of dry mouth, drowsiness, or weight gain. Drawbacks of Nefazodone and Trazodone include the possibility of drowsiness and dizziness.

3. Switch to a different serotonergic medication, e.g. from one SSRI to another SSRI, to an SNRI, or to a non-selective MAO inhibitor. It may be that a different medicine will provide the antidepressant benefits without the sexual problems.

5.3.5 Temporary Augmentation with a Serotonin Antagonist

A "drug holiday" is one way to take a break from the serotonergic effects that cause sexual dysfunction. Another way is to turn off the serotonergic effects chemically, by blocking the serotonin receptors that cause the dysfunction. Some of the tricyclic antidepressants have this effect (see Section 5.3.4), and can be taken on a daily basis for this purpose.

A different approach to is to take a short-lived medication that blocks serotonin receptors (a *serotonin antagonist*). Sexual function should improve during the blockade period. As the medication disappears from the body, the serotonergic effects (both good and bad) return. The allergy medication Cyproheptadine (Periactin) may be used for this purpose.[1]

Cyproheptadine is a combined serotonin and histamine antagonist. It can be effective in alleviating sexual dysfunction, but it has two drawbacks. The first drawback is the usual set of antihistamine side effects, such as drowsiness. The second is that, since it acts to oppose a serotonergic antidepressant, it can suppress any benefits from the antidepressant. Thus undesirable feelings (depression, anxiety, etc.) that have been treated successfully by the antidepressant may also return.

It is important to use a serotonin antagonist only as needed to alleviate sexual dysfunction. Frequent use could render the antidepressant ineffective and negate all of its benefits.

Main Brand Name	Chemical Name	Chemical Type	Half Life	Wash-out Time	On-Label Uses	Off-Label Uses
Periactin	Cypro-heptadine		4 hours	1 day	Allergies; Headache	Sexual Dysfunction (Anti-depressant-induced)

---

[1]Cyproheptadine is also used in the treatment of serotonin syndrome.

5.3.6   Cholinergic Enhancers

A "cholinergic" medication is one that enhances the affects of the neurotransmitter acetylcholine, either by simulating it (as an agonist), or by acting to increase its concentration. Cholinergic medications can reverse problems with muscle weakness (Myasthenia Gravis), control Glaucoma, or treat urinary retention by improving muscular function in the urinary tract.

Neostigmine is a cholinesterase inhibitor that increases acetylcholine concentration by inhibiting the enzyme (acetylcholinesterase) that destroys acetylcholine. It has been used to enhance libido and treat anorgasmia induced by SSRI medications.

Bethanechol has been found useful for treating ED caused by the *anti*-cholinergic effects of many tricyclic antidepressants.

Main Brand Name	Chemical Name	Chemical Type	Half Life	Wash-out Time	On-Label Uses	Off-Label Uses
Prostigmin	Neostigmine		1 hour	5 hours	Myasthenia Gravis	Sexual Dysfunction (Anti-depressant-induced)
Urecholine	Bethanechol		30 minutes	2 hours	Urinary Retention	Sexual Dysfunction (Anti-depressant-induced)

5.3.7   Other Augmentations

The author has heard one anecdotal report that taking the SNRI Reboxetine, along with an SSRI, has alleviated sexual dysfunction due to the latter, although it is not clear why this should be the case.

5.4   Solutions for Problems Caused by Antipsychotics

All antipsychotic medications work by blockading (blocking) the dopamine D_2 receptors in the brain, thus reducing the amount of dopamine-related signaling. (See Chapter 4 for details.) The reduction in dopamine activity alleviates psychosis, but can cause numerous difficulties. This section is concerned specifically with antipsychotic-induced sexual dysfunction, and will not address other undesirable side effects of these medications.

Antipsychotic medications are divided into two categories: "typical" and "atypical" antipsychotics. The older, typical antipsychotics blockade D_2 receptors throughout the brain. The newer, atypical antipsychotics are more selective, and preferentially blockade D2 receptors in the Mesolimbic Dopamine Pathway, which is the area where excess dopamine activity seems to produce the so-called "positive" psychotic symptoms such as hallucinations. The greater specificity of action of the atypical antipsychotics substantially reduces the undesirable side effects (including sexual dysfunction), compared to the typical antipsychotics, but does not eliminate them.

It appears that sexual dysfunction is a side effect that results from blockading D_2 dopamine receptors in the Tuberoinfundibular Dopamine Pathway. Dopamine activity in this pathway controls the rate at which the pituitary gland releases the hormone prolactin. Dopamine blockade in this area causes the pituitary gland to release excess prolactin, which, in sufficiently large amounts, causes hyperprolactinemia. Excess prolactin decreases libido, reducing or eliminating sexual desire. In addition, it can cause reduction in the hormones testosterone and estrogen, negatively affecting libido, erectile function, fertility, bone density in women (osteoporosis), and other aspects of the patient's health.

Treatment of antipsychotic-induced sexual disorder is difficult, as the same neurotransmitter (dopamine) is involved both in libido, and positive psychotic symptoms (such as hallucinations). Simply increasing dopamine activity, in order to alleviate sexual dysfunction, may counteract the benefits of the antipsychotic and trigger psychotic episodes. Thus treatment is largely a balancing act between the needs of the treatment for psychosis on the one hand, and the treatment of suppressed libido on the other. (See www.medsafe.govt.nz/Profs/PUarticles/hyperpro.htm for a good description of the issues involved)

The treatment strategies for antipsychotic-induced sexual dysfunction are essentially a subset of those for antidepressant-induced sexual dysfunction, except that "antidepressant" is replaced by "antipsychotic." The relevant strategies will not be repeated here in detail, but are listed below:

- Change the time of the dose (Section 5.3.1).

- Change the size of the dose (Section 5.3.3).

- Change the medication, especially from a typical to an atypical antipsychotic.

- Treat endocrine problems such as low testosterone or estrogen with hormone-replacement therapy (Section 5.1.2.1).

- Reduce prolactin production with a dopamine agonist, but be careful not to counteract the benefits of the antipsychotic medication in the process (Section 5.1.2.2).

More research is needed to find better ways to treat sexual dysfunction caused by antipsychotic medications.

5.5 Conclusion

The bad news is that medications taken to improve mental health may degrade sexual health. The good news is that, for many people, effective remedies for sexual dysfunction do exist. Much as is the case with antidepressants taken for depression, one may have to try several of the existing remedies for sexual dysfunction in order to find one that works satisfactorily. In this matter, as is so often the case with psychotropic medications, patience is as much a necessity as a virtue.

Chapter 6

Glossary

These terms are often encountered in descriptions of psychotropic medications and mental illness.

Adjunctive Therapy. The use of a medication to treat a problem in combination with some other medication also prescribed for that problem.

Adrenergic. An *adrenergic* medication is one that increases the concentration or activity of the hormone epinephrine. The term comes from the word *adrenaline*, which is an alternate name for epinephrine. Epinephrine is closely related to the neurotransmitter norepinephrine.

Affect. A general term for emotion, often in reference to body language and facial expressions that indicate the emotion. *Flattened affect*, or *blunted affect*, refers to the impairment or absence of the normal range of emotion.

Agonist. A chemical that simulates or amplifies the effects of another chemical. The effect of taking, say, a dopamine agonist is similar to increasing the concentration of dopamine in the brain. In essence, an agonist may serve as a substitute for the other chemical.

Agranulocytosis. A condition in which the count of white blood cells is low, which increases the susceptibility to infection.

Akathisia. Motor restlessness, including quivering and an inability to sit still. In severe cases, akathisia makes resting and sleeping impossible. (Section 4.4.3)

Alzheimer's Disease. A progressive brain disorder that causes dementia. The dementia produced by Alzheimer's disease is a result of the gradual destruction of brain tissue due to the accumulation of abnormal protein structures known as amyloid plaques.

Anergia. Lack of energy.

Anhedonia. The inability to feel pleasure (a typical symptom of depression), where "pleasure" refers not simply to physical sensations, but any positive emotions (happiness, joy, satisfaction, fulfillment, etc.)

Anorgasmia. Difficulty in achieving orgasm.

Anosognosia. Impaired ability, or inability, to recognize or believe that one is ill. People who have anosognosia often refuse to take medication for their illness, believing it either unnecessary, or an attempt to harm or control them. (Chapter 4)

Antagonist. A chemical that suppresses the effects of another chemical. The effect of taking, say, a dopamine antagonist is similar to decreasing the concentration of dopamine in the brain.

Aplastic Anemia. A group of related disorders characterized by the failure of bone marrow to produce all three types of blood cells: Red blood cells, white blood cells, and platelets. The symptoms include unexplained infections, unexpected bleeding, and fatigue (due to insufficient white blood cells, platelets, and red blood cells). The condition is diagnosed by measuring the blood-cell concentration, or reduction in the number of cells in the bone marrow (from blood or marrow samples, respectively).

Attention Deficit Hyperactivity Disorder (ADHD). A disorder, which is diagnosed primarily among children, characterized by inability to pay attention or focus on tasks at hand (such as schoolwork), hyperactive physical behavior (fidgeting, extreme restlessness), and difficulty controlling impulsive behavior.

Bipolar Disorder. An illness in which manic and depressive episodes alternate. This illness was formerly called *Manic-Depressive Disorder*. (Chapter 3)

Blockade. The action of certain medications to decrease the level of signalling associated with a particular neurotransmitter, by binding to, and blocking, receptors associated with that neurotransmitter. *Dopamine blockade*, for example, is the primary mechanism of antipsychotic medications (Section 4.1.1)

Catatonia. A psychiatric condition most commonly described as a state of stupor. The stupor type of catatonia is an apathetic state, and often physically frozen or rigid state, in which the person is either oblivious to, or does not react to, external stimuli (such as attempts to communicate). A second type of catatonia, known as catatonic excitement, is characterized by constant agitation and excitation, a type of hyperactivity that is also purposeless.

Central Nervous System (CNS). The brain and spinal cord.

Cyclothymic Disorder. A mild form of bipolar disorder. (Chapter 3)

Delusion. A false belief; i.e., a belief that is contrary to observed fact, or extremely unrealistic. (Chapter 4)

Dementia. Dementia is the name for a collection of symptoms having to do with the deterioration of mental function; namely, the progressive decline in memory, attention span, and the ability to learn, reason, make judgments, and communicate. Dementia can be produced by a variety of neurological disorders, such as Alzheimer's disease.

Depression. A persistent mood characterized by sadness, inability to feel pleasure, and other unpleasant feelings. (Chapter 2)

Depressive Episode. A period of time during which a person's mood is characterized by depression.

Diabetes. An illness in which blood glucose (sugar) levels are above normal, because of an inability to metabolize glucose. The latter problem is due to insufficient production or utilization of insulin, the hormone responsible for metabolizing glucose. Diabetes is a very serious illness, which can rapidly lead to death if untreated. Treatment consists of careful diet, insulin injections, and medications to control blood-sugar levels.

Dopamine. A neurotransmitter. (Section 1.3.1)

Dopamine Agonist(DA). A chemical that acts as a substitute for dopamine. (Section 2.7)

Dopamine Reuptake Inhibitor (DRI). An antidepressant that increases the concentration of dopamine. (Section 2.5.10)

Double Depression Major Depression experienced on top of dysthymia.

Dysthymia. Mild chronic depression, which is not episodic, but remains steady over time.

Dystonia. Any sustained and involuntary contraction of the muscles, which leads to twisted and distorted posture. (Section 4.4.3)

Electroconvulsive Therapy (ECT). A technique for treating depression, bipolar disorder, schizophrenia, and catatonia. External electrodes are used to stimulate parts of the brain with an electric current, in order to trigger seizures that alleviate the symptoms of these illnesses. (Section 1.7.2)

EIAED Enzyme-Inducing Anti-Epileptic Drug. This is a category of medication used in the treatment of seizures and bipolar disorder, so named because they cause the liver to increase production of the CYP450 enzyme. (Section 3.6)

ED Erectile dysfunction.

Endogenous Depression. A state of depression for which there is no apparent precipitating cause.

Extrapyramidal Symptoms (EPS). Any of a variety of movement disorders, including Parkinsonism, Dystonia, Akathisia, and Tardive Dyskinesia. These disorders are often induced by medication that suppress dopamine activity in the Extrapyramidal System, such as antipsychotics (see Section 4.4.3). The Extrapyramidal System is part of the brain's motor system, and is involved in the coordination of movement.

Erectile Dysfunction (ED). Difficulty achieving or maintaining a satisfactory erection. (Chapter 5)

-ergic. (As in dopaminergic, serotonergic, GABA-ergic). A medication is said to be XXX-ergic if it increases the concentration of XXX, or has an effect on the brain and body similar to what an increase in XXX would have. (The term is often used to refer to side effects of medications, e.g., "serotonergic effects such as decrease of libido," "anticholinergic effects such as low blood pressure," etc.)

Food and Drug Administration (FDA). The United States government agency responsible for approving medications for prescription use.

Gamma Aminobutyric Acid (GABA). A neurotransmitter. (Section 1.3.2, and Section 3.2)

GABA Analog (GA). A chemical that increases the concentration or effects of the neurotransmitter GABA. GABA analogs are used to treat bipolar disorder. (Section 3.7)

GABA Reuptake Inhibitor (GRI). A mood stabilizer that increases the concentration of GABA. (Section 3.7)

Glutamate. A neurotransmitter. (Section 1.3.3)

Half Life. The time required for the body to eliminate (metabolize or expel) half of the total amount of the medication it currently contains.

Hallucination. Any subjective sensory perception that does not arise from an external stimulus, such as voices or images that are not actually present. Hallucinations may involve any of the senses, and be simple (e.g., a taste) or complex (e.g., complete conversations). (Chapter 4)

Hyperprolactinemia. A disorder characterized by excess amounts of the hormone prolactin in the blood. Excess prolactin can cause a variety of symptoms, including depression, sexual dysfunction, and loss of libido. Women may have a variety of menstrual problems, infertility, hirsutism, or obesity. Men may have low, or no, sperm production. The major causes of hyperprolactinemia are pituitary-gland tumors, hypothyroidism, hypothalamic disease, chronic kidney failure, cirrhosis, and antipsychotic medications.

Hypertension. High blood pressure, which is high enough to be a health risk.

Hypertensive Crisis. A sudden, dramatic increase in blood pressure, great enough to be dangerous. A hypertensive crisis may cause discomfort, severe headache, permanent injury, or even death.

Hypoactive Sexual Desire (HSD). Also known as *low libido*, or *Inadequate Sexual Desire (ISD)*, this term refers to the condition of having a level of sexual desire that is low enough to be considered a problem by the person or couple affected.

Hypomania. A milder form of mania, typically of shorter duration, which is characterized primarily by euphoria or irritability.

Hyponatremia. Low sodium concentration in the blood. This condition most commonly occurs when people are doing strenuous work in hot environments, where they lose a great deal of salt through perspiration. but don't replace it by consuming enough salt in the diet. When low in sodium, the brain cells absorb too much water, and the brain swells, pushing against the skull. The condition can cause nausea, vomiting, fatigue, dulled thinking, clumsiness, seizures, coma, and even death. It is very serious, but also easily treatable.

Hypotension. Low blood pressure, which may cause dizziness or fainting. *Orthostatic hypotension* refers to a sudden decrease in blood pressure when rising after sitting or lying down.

Libido. The capacity for sexual desire.

Major Depression, or Major Depressive Disorder. Severe depression, which may be episodic, last for weeks or months, and recur after months or years. (Chapter 2)

Mania. A mood characterized by excess, as in some combination of the following: Excessive energy, excessively rapid speech or thinking, excessive elation, excessive self-confidence (leading to poor judgment and grandiose plans), excessive wakefulness, and excessive elation, irritability, or anger. (Chapter 3)

Manic-Depressive Disorder. The obsolete name for what is now called bipolar disorder.

Manic Episode. A period of time during which a person's mood is characterized by mania.

Metabolite. A chemical produced by the metabolic transformation (metabolization) of another chemical. *Metabolite* is the opposite of precursor. If chemical A is metabolized to produce chemical B, then A is a precursor of B, and B is a metabolite of A.

Monoamine Oxidase. A family of enzymes (chemicals that break down other chemicals) that metabolize (destroy) neurotransmitters. (Section 2.4)

Monoamine Oxidase Inhibitor (MAOI). An antidepressant that works by disabling monoamine oxidase molecules. (Section 2.4)

Monotherapy. The use of a single medication to treat a medical problem.

Neuralgia. Pain, intermittent or steady, often severe, extending along a nerve or group of nerves.

Neuroleptic. A medication that blockades the dopamine D_2 receptor. The word essentially means "calming," but the primary use of these medications is in the treatment of psychosis, arising from schizophrenia or other conditions. When used in the context of treating psychosis, neuroleptic is an outdated term, and the term *antipsychotic* is preferred in current usage. However, the term neuroleptic applies to medications that have this mechanism but are used for purposes other than the treatment of psychosis, such as the control of serious vomiting.

Neuroleptic Malignant Syndrome (NMS). A rare, but life threatening reaction to neuroleptic (anti-psychotic) medication, consisting of fever, muscular rigidity, altered mental status, and dysfunction of the autonomic nervous system. Much less common than tardive dyskinesia. (Section 4.3.3 and www.emedicine.com)

Neuron. An impulse- (signal-) conducting cell. The brain, spinal column, and nerves are comprised of neurons. (Section 1.3)

Neurotransmitter. A chemical that conveys a signal from one neuron to another, by propagating across a synaptic gap. Many types of neurotransmitters are known. (Section 1.3)

Noradrenergic. A *noradrenergic* medication is one that increases the concentration or activity of the neurotransmitter norepinephrine. The terms comes from the word *noradrenalin*, which is an alternate name for norepinephrine. Norepinephrine is closely related to the hormone epinephrine.

Noradrenergic/Specific Serotonergic Antidepressan (NaSSA). An antidepressant that increases the release of norepinephrine and serotonin. (Section 2.5.8)

Norepinephrine. A neurotransmitter. (Section 1.3.4)

Norepinephrine-Dopamine Reuptake Inhibitor (NDRI). An antidepressant that increases the concentration of both norepinephrine and dopamine. (Section 2.5.7)

Norepinephrine Reuptake Inhibitor (NRI). A medication that increases the concentration of norepinephrine, used to treat ADHD and depression. (Section 2.5.6)

Off-Label, On-Label. The *on-label* uses of a medication are those which the FDA (Food and Drug Administration of the United States) has officially approved, meaning for which it has found the medication to be effective. The *off-label* uses are any for which the FDA has not declared a medication to be effective. The lack of FDA approval doesn't mean the medication doesn't work for off-label conditions; it simply means that the FDA hasn't issued an official finding supporting the effectiveness of the medication for those uses. Off-label uses of psychotropic medications are common, and not infrequently lead to subsequent FDA-approved studies and approvals. The use of anticonvulsive medications to treat bipolar disorder is a good example of migration from off-label to on-label status.

Paranoia. Extreme distrust of others, to the point of believing that others are trying to harm or control one. (Chapter 4)

Parkinsonism. A condition, often induced by antipsychotic medications, whose symptoms resemble those of Parkinson's disease (Section 4.4.3). Symptoms include muscular rigidity, tremor, and impaired motor control (i.e., difficulty grasping and manipulating objects, walking in a straight line, and so forth).

Parkinson's Disease. A chronic, and progressive, disease of the Central Nervous System, in which the brain cells that produce dopamine gradually die off. The steady reduction in dopamine levels in the brain leads to steady worsening of the symptoms, namely tremors, muscle stiffness, slowness of movement, poor balance and coordiation, depression, sleeping, and numerous other problems.

Pathway. A pathway in the brain is is a bundle of nerve fibers that follow a particular path, often associated with the activity of a particular neurotransmitter.

Precursor. A chemical that is converted into another chemical of interest. A serotonin precursor, for example, is a chemical that is converted (at least partially) into serotonin. *Precursor* is the opposite of metabolite. If chemical A is metabolized to produce chemical B, then A is a precursor of B, and B is a metabolite of A.

Priapism. For men only. A sustained and dangerous erection that can last for a day or more. It constitutes a medical emergency, and must be treated quickly by medication or surgery, to avoid permanent damage to the penis.

Psychopharmacology. The study of medications used to treat different kinds of mental illness.

Psychosis. An extremely serious mental illness characterized by one or more of the following: visual, auditory, or olfactory hallucinations; delusions (beliefs that clearly contradict reality); inability to think coherently; and inability to realize that one has any of these problems (anosognosia). People suffering from psychosis are described as *psychotic*, and may have discussions with people who don't exist, and exhibit bizarre and irrational behavior, including verbal and (rarely) physical violence. Types of psychotic disorders (psychoses) include Schizophrenia, Schizoaffective Disorder, Delusional or Paranoid Disorder, and Psychotic Depression. (Chapter 4)

Psychotropic. A medication that affects the functioning of the brain, often by modifying neurotransmitter chemistry.

QT Interval. The duration of electrical activity that controls contraction of the heart muscle. The QT interval is measured by an EKG device.

QT Prolongation Prolongation of the QT interval by medication, such as the typical antipsychotics, which can cause a serious heart-rhythm problem called Torsades de Pointes. The latter condition can cause fainting or death. (See www.arizonacert.org and Section 4.3.4 for details.)

Receptor. A receptor is a localized region on the surface of a neuron that receives a signal from another neuron (in the form of a pulse of neurotransmitter molecules squirted across the synaptic gap between the neurons), and initiates some activity in the receiving neuron. Each receptor responds to a particular neurotransmitter, and there are usually multiple sub-types of receptor for each neurotransmitter. (Section 1.3)

Reversible MAO Inhibitor (RIMA). A type of MAO inhibitor that does not disable the enzyme monoamine oxidase permanently. The disabling reaction is reversible, a characteristic that reduces problems with food and drug interactions.

Schizophrenia. An illness characterised by psychosis (a collection of symptoms that includes hallucinations, delusions, and anosognosia), cognitive impairment, and inability to feel pleasure or satisfaction. (Chapter 4)

Serotonin. A neurotransmitter. (Section 1.3.5)

Serotonin Agonist/Reuptake Inhibitor (SARI). An antidepressant that increases the concentration of serotonin, and promotes the conversion of the serotonin precursor 5HT to serotonin. (Section 2.5.4)

Serotonin/Norepinephrine Reuptake Inhibitor (SNRI). An antidepressant that increases the concentration of both serotonin and norepinephrine. (Section 2.5.5)

Serotonin Reuptake Accelerator (SRA). An antidepressant that decreases the concentration of serotonin. (Section 2.5.9)

Selective Serotonin Reuptake Inhibitor (SSRI). An antidepressant that increases the concentration of serotonin. (Section 2.5.3)

Serotonin Syndrome. A condition resulting from excessive levels of serotonin, caused by taking an excess of medications that increase serotonin concentration. The condition is characterized by the presence of at least one abnormal symptom in each of these three categories: disturbance of mental status (anxiety, agitation, confusion, restlessness, hypomania, hallucinations and coma); motor changes (tremor, involuntary twitching, loss of coordination, and muscle tightness and stiffness, especially in the legs); and disturbance of the autonomic nervous system (fever, sweating, nausea, vomiting, diarrhea and hypertension). Life-threatening complications include coma, seizures, blood coagulation, and breakdown of muscle tissue, which can cause kidney damage. While Serotonin Syndrome can be very dangerous, and must be treated promptly by a physician, most cases that occur are mild, and quickly disappear when the offending medication is halted. Benzodiazepines (excluding Clonazepam), as in Section 3.9, may be used to relieve the symptoms. More severe cases can be treated with serotonin antagonists such as Cyproheptadine (Section 5.3.5), methysergide, and beta blockers such as Propranolol. (Section 2.2.4)

Sexual Dysfunction. Any problem that impairs or prevents satisfactory sexual functioning. (Chapter 5)

Somatoform Disorder. A condition characterized by a variety of physical symptoms, typically lasting for several years, that cannot be attributed to other illnesses. Symptoms include frequent headaches, back pain, abdominal cramping and pelvic pain, pain in the joints, legs and arms, chest or abdominal pain, gastrointestinal problems (nausea, bloating, vomiting, diarrhea and food intolerance), painful urination, and sexual dysfunction. Somatoform disorder is difficult to diagnose, because its symptoms are similar to many other illnesses. Its cause is not known, but may be related to abnormalities of signal propagation in the nervous system.

Stevens-Johnson Syndrome. An allergic reaction to medication characterized by painful blistering of the mucous membranes (e.g. in and around the mouth, throat, anus, genitals, vagina, and eyes), and patchy areas of rash, often preceded by flu-like symptoms and high fever. Blistered skin peels off very easily. This illness is very serious, and can be fatal.

Synapse, or Synaptic Gap. The gap between the signal-transmitting region (an axon terminal) of one neuron, and the signal-receiving portion (receptors) of an adjacent neuron. (Section 1.3)

Tardive Dyskinesia (TD). Involuntary movements of the tongue, lips, face, upper body, and extremities. Although the condition may occur naturally, it most often occurs as a result of treatment with neuroleptic (anti-psychotic) medications (e.g., dopamine antagonists). It is a very serious condition, which may or may not go away when medication is stopped. It is a principle risk in the use of antipsychotic medications. (Section 4.3.1 and www.emedicine.com)

Tricyclic Antidepressant (TCA). An antidepressant medication that increases the concentration norepinephrine and serotonin, named for the tricyclic chemical structure shared by members of this family (although one such medication, Maprotiline, actually has a tetracyclic structure). (Section 2.5.2)

Torsades de Pointes. A type of cardiac arrhythmia (abnormal heartbeat) that can cause fainting or death. It can be caused by medications that prolong the QT interval, such as the typical antipsychotics. (Section 4.3.4 and www.arizonacert.org)

Tourette's Disorder. A neurological disorder, characterized by involuntary movements, and vocal outbursts (known as *tics*), which have persisted for at least 12 months.

Toxic Epidermal Necrolysis. An allergic reaction to medication, very similar to Stevens-Johnson Syndrome, with the additional symptom that large areas of skin may blister and peel off (even 30% or more of the skin, in many cases). This illness is very serious, and can be fatal.

Transcranial Magnetic Stimulation (TMS). A technique for treating depression by stimulating parts of the brain with time-varying, externally-generated magnetic-fields. It is also abbreviated as "rTMS," for repetitive TMS. (Section 2.2.2)

Transdermal. A skin patch. This is a plastic patch, coated with adhesive on one side, which sticks to the skin. The medication stored in the patch flows slowly through the skin into the blood stream.

Tyramine. A common amino acid, found in food and in the body, which affects blood pressure. An excess of tyramine causes high blood pressure, and associated symptoms such as headaches. A sufficiently large excess can cause a dangerous hypertensive crisis. The digestive tract normally eliminates excess tyramine by destroying it with the enzyme Monoamine Oxidase A(MAO-A). Medications that inhibit MAO-A impair this regulatory mechanism, and consumption of tyramine while taking these medications can produce a hypertensive crisis.

Common foods that contain high levels of tyramine include aged cheeses, any aged or preserved meats (bacon, sausage), red wines, miso soup, brewer's yeast, and most yeast-containing products. Baker's yeast, used to make bread and other leavened foods, does not contain tyramine.

Tyramine accumulates naturally in foods as they age. Aged foods of any kind, including refrigerated leftovers more than a day old, may contain high levels of tyramine.

Unipolar Depression. A synonym for depression, used to distinguish it from the depressive episodes of bipolar disorder.

Vagus Nerve Stimulation (VNS). A technique for treating seizure disorders and depression by electrically stimulating the Vagus Nerve. (Section 2.2.1)

Vesicle. A chamber in a neuron, which stores neurotransmitter molecules. Some neurotransmitters are synthesized inside vesicles, while others are synthesized elsewhere in the neuron, and piped into vesicles for storage. (Section 1.3)

Washout Time. The time from termination of medication until another, potentially conflicting one can be used; or, equivalently, the time from termination until the medication is effectively gone from the body. Often taken to be five half-lives.

Chapter 7

Medication Index

The medication index shows where to find each medication described in this book. Each medication has both a chemical name, and a principal brand name by which it is most often (or originally) known.

Many medications have alternate brand names as well, often varying from country to country. Principal brand names appear in **bold** type in the index, while chemical names appear in *italics*, and other brand names appear in regular type.

Names are in alphabetical order, with any leading numbers or other non-alphabetic characters shown in the name, but ignored for sorting purposes.

Aiglonyl (**Dolmatil**, or *Sulpiride*) 108
Alboral (**Valium**, or *Diazepam*) 83
Aldazine (**Mellaril**, or *Thioridazine*) 100
ALDO (**Haldol**, or *Haloperidol*) 101
Alimoral (**Dolmatil**, or *Sulpiride*) 108
Aliseum (**Valium**, or *Diazepam*) 83
Allegron (**Pamelor**, or *Nortriptyline*) 43
Allodene (**Dexedrine**, or *Dextroamphetamine*) 63
Almazine (**Ativan**, or *Lorazepam*) 83
Aloperidin (**Haldol**, or *Haloperidol*) 101
Aloperidol (**Haldol**, or *Haloperidol*) 101
Aloperidolo (**Haldol**, or *Haloperidol*) 101
Aloperidon (**Haldol**, or *Haloperidol*) 101
Alpha-Chlorprothixene (**Truxal**, or *Chlorprothixene*) 101
Alpha-Methylbenzeneethaneamine (**Dexedrine**, or *Dextroamphetamine*) 63
Alplax (**Xanax**, or *Alprazolam*) 83
Alprazolam (**Xanax**) 83
Alpronax (**Xanax**, or *Alprazolam*) 83
Alprostadil (**Muse**) 114
Alprostadil Prostoglandin E1 (**Muse**, or *Alprostadil*) 114
Alti-Bromocriptine (**Parlodel**, or *Bromocriptine*) 59
Alti-Valproic (**Depakene**, or *Valproic Acid*) 75
Altilev (**Pamelor**, or *Nortriptyline*) 43
Alupram (**Valium**, or *Diazepam*) 83
Alviz (**Xanax**, or *Alprazolam*) 83
Alzapam (**Ativan**, or *Lorazepam*) 83
Amantadine (**Symmetrel**) 59
Amantidine (**Symmetrel**, or *Amantadine*) 59
Amidopropyldimethylbetaine (**Urecholine**, or *Bethanechol*) 123
Amimetilina (**Vivactil**, or *Protriptyline*) 43
Aminazin (**Thorazine**, or *Chlorpromazine*) 100
Aminazine (**Thorazine**, or *Chlorpromazine*) 100
Amineptine (**Survector**) 56
Aminoadamantane (**Symmetrel**, or *Amantadine*) 59
Amiprol (**Valium**, or *Diazepam*) 83
Amisulpride (**Solian**) 108
Amitid (**Elavil**, or *Amitriptyline*) 43
Amitril (**Elavil**, or *Amitriptyline*) 43
Amitrip (**Elavil**, or *Amitriptyline*) 43
Amitriptyline (**Elavil**) 43
Amitriprolidine (**Elavil**, or *Amitriptyline*) 43
Amitriptylin (**Elavil**, or *Amitriptyline*) 43
Amitryptiline (**Elavil**, or *Amitriptyline*) 43

Amitryptyline (**Elavil**, or *Amitriptyline*) 43

Amoxapine (**Asendin**) 43

Amoxepine (**Asendin**, or *Amoxapine*) 43

Ampazine (**Sparine**, or *Promazine*) 100

Amphetamine (mixture) (**Adderall**) 63

Amphetamine (**Dexedrine**, or *Dextroamphetamine*) 63

Ampliactil (**Thorazine**, or *Chlorpromazine*) 100

Amytriptiline (**Elavil**, or *Amitriptyline*) 43

An-Ding (**Valium**, or *Diazepam*) 83

Anafranil (*Clomipramine*) 43

Anatensol (**Prolixin Injection**, or *Fluphenazine Decanoate*) 100

Aneural (**Ludiomil**, or *Maprotiline*) 43

Animex-On (**Prozac**, or *Fluoxetine*) 47

Anorexide (**Dexedrine**, or *Dextroamphetamine*) 63

Anorexine (**Dexedrine**, or *Dextroamphetamine*) 63

Ansial (**BuSpar**, or *Buspirone*) 119

Ansiced (**BuSpar**, or *Buspirone*) 119

Ansilan (**Prozac**, or *Fluoxetine*) 47

Ansiolin (**Valium**, or *Diazepam*) 83

Ansiolisina (**Valium**, or *Diazepam*) 83

Antelepsin (**Klonopin**, or *Clonazepam*) 83

Antideprin (**Tofranil**, or *Imipramine*) 43

Antilepsin (**Klonopin**, or *Clonazepam*) 83

Anxiedin (**Ativan**, or *Lorazepam*) 83

Anxiron (**BuSpar**, or *Buspirone*) 119

Apaurin (**Valium**, or *Diazepam*) 83

Aphrodyne (**Yocon**, or *Yohimbine*) 116

Aplacassee (**Ativan**, or *Lorazepam*) 83

Apo Peram Tab (**Trilafon**, or *Perphenazine*) 100

Apo-Amitriptyline (**Elavil**, or *Amitriptyline*) 43

Apo-Bromocriptine (**Parlodel**, or *Bromocriptine*) 59

Apo-Carbamazepine (**Tegretol**, or *Carbamazepine*) 77

Apo-Chlordiazepoxide (**Librium**, or *Chlordiazepoxide*) 83

Apo-Diazepam (**Valium**, or *Diazepam*) 83

Apo-Fluphenazine (**Prolixin Injection**, or *Fluphenazine Decanoate*) 100

Apo-Haloperidol (**Haldol**, or *Haloperidol*) 101

Apo-Imipramine (**Tofranil**, or *Imipramine*) 43

Apo-Perphenazine (**Trilafon**, or *Perphenazine*) 100

Apo-Selegiline (**Eldepryl**, or *Selegiline (oral)*) 37

Apo-Sertraline (**Zoloft**, or *Sertraline*) 47

Apo-Trifluoperazine (**Stelazine**, or *Trifluoperazine*) 100

Apo-Trimip (**Vivactil**, or *Protriptyline*) 43

Apokyn (**Uprima**, or *Apomorphine*) 115

Benzolone (**Dexedrine**, or *Dextroamphetamine*) 63

Berkomine (**Tofranil**, or *Imipramine*) 43

Berophen (**Sparine**, or *Promazine*) 100

Besacholine (**Urecholine**, or *Bethanechol*) 123

Bespar (**BuSpar**, or *Buspirone*) 119

Bestrol (**Xanax**, or *Alprazolam*) 83

Beta-Aminopropylbenzene (**Dexedrine**, or *Dextroamphetamine*) 63

Beta-Methyl Carbachol Chloride (**Urecholine**, or *Bethanechol*) 123

Beta-Methylimipramine (**Surmontil**, or *Trimipramine*) 43

Beta-phenylethylhydrazine (**Nardil**, or *Phenelzine*) 39

(+/-)-beta-Phenylisopropylamine (**Dexedrine**, or *Dextroamphetamine*) 63

Betanamin (**Cylert**, or *Pemoline*) 63

Bethaine Choline Chloride (**Urecholine**, or *Bethanechol*) 123

Bethanechol (**Urecholine**) 123

Bethanechol Chloride (**Urecholine**, or *Bethanechol*) 123

Bialzepam (**Valium**, or *Diazepam*) 83

Bimaran (**Desyrel**, or *Trazodone*) 49

Bioperidolo (**Haldol**, or *Haloperidol*) 101

Biston (**Tegretol**, or *Carbamazepine*) 77

BMIH (**Marplan**, or *Isocarboxazid*) 39

Bonatranquan (**Ativan**, or *Lorazepam*) 83

Bromergocryptine (**Parlodel**, or *Bromocriptine*) 59

Bromocriptine (**Parlodel**) 59

Bromocriptin (**Parlodel**, or *Bromocriptine*) 59

Bromocriptina (**Parlodel**, or *Bromocriptine*) 59

Bromocriptinum (**Parlodel**, or *Bromocriptine*) 59

Bromocryptine (**Parlodel**, or *Bromocriptine*) 59

Bromoergocriptine (**Parlodel**, or *Bromocriptine*) 59

Bromoergocryptine (**Parlodel**, or *Bromocriptine*) 59

Brotopon (**Haldol**, or *Haloperidol*) 101

Bruceine D (**Depakene**, or *Valproic Acid*) 75

BTC (**Urecholine**, or *Bethanechol*) 123

Buccastem (**Compazine**, or *Prochlorperazine*) 100

Bupropion (**Wellbutrin**) 53

BuSpar (*Buspirone*) 119

Buspimen (**BuSpar**, or *Buspirone*) 119

Buspinol (**BuSpar**, or *Buspirone*) 119

Buspirona (**BuSpar**, or *Buspirone*) 119

Buspirone (**BuSpar**) 119

Buspironum (**BuSpar**, or *Buspirone*) 119

Buspisal (**BuSpar**, or *Buspirone*) 119

Cabaser (**Dostinex**, or *Cabergoline*) 59

Cabergoline (**Dostinex**) 59

Cabergolina (**Dostinex**, or *Cabergoline*) 59

Cabergolinum (**Dostinex**, or *Cabergoline*) 59

Calepsin (**Tegretol**, or *Carbamazepine*) 77

Calmocitene (**Valium**, or *Diazepam*) 83

Calmoflorine (**Dolmatil**, or *Sulpiride*) 108

Calmpose (**Valium**, or *Diazepam*) 83

Calocain (**Ritalin**, or *Methylphenidate*) 63

Calodal (**Serentil**, or *Mesoridazine*) 100

Camapine (**Tegretol**, or *Carbamazepine*) 77

Camcolit (**Lithobid**, or *Lithium Carbonate*) 73

Capazine (**Compazine**, or *Prochlorperazine*) 100

Carbamazepine (**Tegretol**) 77

Carbadac (**Tegretol**, or *Carbamazepine*) 77

Carbamazepen (**Tegretol**, or *Carbamazepine*) 77

Carbamezepine (**Tegretol**, or *Carbamazepine*) 77

Carbamylmethylcholine Chloride (**Urecholine**, or *Bethanechol*) 123

Carbatol (**Tegretol**, or *Carbamazepine*) 77

Carbatrol (**Tegretol**, or *Carbamazepine*) 77

Carbazene (**Tegretol**, or *Carbamazepine*) 77

Carbazep (**Tegretol**, or *Carbamazepine*) 77

Carbazepine (**Tegretol**, or *Carbamazepine*) 77

Carbazina (**Tegretol**, or *Carbamazepine*) 77

Carbelan (**Tegretol**, or *Carbamazepine*) 77

Carbex (**Eldepryl**, or *Selegiline (oral)*) 37

Carbium (**Tegretol**, or *Carbamazepine*) 77

Carbolit (**Lithobid**, or *Lithium Carbonate*) 73

Carbolith (**Lithobid**, or *Lithium Carbonate*) 73

Carbolithium (**Lithobid**, or *Lithium Carbonate*) 73

Carmaz (**Tegretol**, or *Carbamazepine*) 77

Carpaz (**Tegretol**, or *Carbamazepine*) 77

Carzepin (**Tegretol**, or *Carbamazepine*) 77

Carzepine (**Tegretol**, or *Carbamazepine*) 77

Cassadan (**Xanax**, or *Alprazolam*) 83

Caverject (**Muse**, or *Alprostadil*) 114

CD 2 (**Librium**, or *Chlordiazepoxide*) 83

CDO (**Librium**, or *Chlordiazepoxide*) 83

CDP (**Librium**, or *Chlordiazepoxide*) 83

Ceglution (**Lithobid**, or *Lithium Carbonate*) 73

Ceglution 300 (**Lithobid**, or *Lithium Carbonate*) 73

Celexa (*Citalopram*) 47

Censpar (**BuSpar**, or *Buspirone*) 119

Censtim (**Tofranil**, or *Imipramine*) 43

Censtin (**Tofranil**, or *Imipramine*) 43

Centedein (**Ritalin**, or *Methylphenidate*) 63
Centedrin (**Ritalin**, or *Methylphenidate*) 63
Centedrine (**Ritalin**, or *Methylphenidate*) 63
Centramin (**Cylert**, or *Pemoline*) 63
Centredin (**Ritalin**, or *Methylphenidate*) 63
Cercine (**Valium**, or *Diazepam*) 83
Ceregulart (**Valium**, or *Diazepam*) 83
Championyl (**Dolmatil**, or *Sulpiride*) 108
Chlonazepam (**Klonopin**, or *Clonazepam*) 83
Chlorpromazine (**Thorazine**) 100
Chloradiazepoxide (**Librium**, or *Chlordiazepoxide*) 83
Chlorazepate (**Tranxene**, or *Clorazepate*) 83
Chlorazepic acid (**Tranxene**, or *Clorazepate*) 83
Chlordelazin (**Thorazine**, or *Chlorpromazine*) 100
Chlorderazin (**Thorazine**, or *Chlorpromazine*) 100
Chlordiazepoxide (**Librium**) 83
Chlordiazachel (**Librium**, or *Chlordiazepoxide*) 83
Chlordiazepoxid (**Librium**, or *Chlordiazepoxide*) 83
Chlordiazepoxide Base (**Librium**, or *Chlordiazepoxide*) 83
Chlordiazepoxidum (**Librium**, or *Chlordiazepoxide*) 83
Chloridazepoxide (**Librium**, or *Chlordiazepoxide*) 83
Chloridiazepide (**Librium**, or *Chlordiazepoxide*) 83
Chloridiazepoxide (**Librium**, or *Chlordiazepoxide*) 83
Chlorimipramine (**Anafranil**, or *Clomipramine*) 43
Chlormeprazine (**Compazine**, or *Prochlorperazine*) 100
Chlorodiazepoxide (**Librium**, or *Chlordiazepoxide*) 83
3-Chloroimipramine (**Anafranil**, or *Clomipramine*) 43
Chloroprothixene (**Truxal**, or *Chlorprothixene*) 101
Chlorperazine (**Compazine**, or *Prochlorperazine*) 100
Chlorperphenazine (**Trilafon**, or *Perphenazine*) 100
Chlorprothixene (**Truxal**) 101
Chlorpromados (**Thorazine**, or *Chlorpromazine*) 100
Chlorpromanyl (**Thorazine**, or *Chlorpromazine*) 100
Chlorprothixen (**Truxal**, or *Chlorprothixene*) 101
Chlorprothixine (**Truxal**, or *Chlorprothixene*) 101
Chlorprotixen (**Truxal**, or *Chlorprothixene*) 101
Chlorprotixene (**Truxal**, or *Chlorprothixene*) 101
Chlorprotixine (**Truxal**, or *Chlorprothixene*) 101
Chlothixen (**Truxal**, or *Chlorprothixene*) 101
Chlozepid (**Librium**, or *Chlordiazepoxide*) 83
CIA (**Cialis**, or *Tadalafil*) 114
Cialis (*Tadalafil*) 114
Cialis/Tadalafil Hcl (**Cialis**, or *Tadalafil*) 114

Cialis/Taladafil (**Cialis**, or *Tadalafil*) 114
4311/B Ciba (**Ritalin**, or *Methylphenidate*) 63
Cipralex (**Lexapro**, or *Escitalopram*) 47
Cipram (**Celexa**, or *Citalopram*) 47
Cipramil (**Celexa**, or *Citalopram*) 47
Cis-Chlorprothixene (**Truxal**, or *Chlorprothixene*) 101
Citalopram (**Celexa**) 47
Citalopramum (**Celexa**, or *Citalopram*) 47
Cloazepam (**Klonopin**, or *Clonazepam*) 83
Clofranil (**Anafranil**, or *Clomipramine*) 43
Clomifril (**Anafranil**, or *Clomipramine*) 43
Clomipramine (**Anafranil**) 43
Clomipramina (**Anafranil**, or *Clomipramine*) 43
Clomipraminum (**Anafranil**, or *Clomipramine*) 43
Clonazepam (**Klonopin**) 83
Clonazepamum (**Klonopin**, or *Clonazepam*) 83
Clonopin (**Klonopin**, or *Clonazepam*) 83
Clopoxide (**Librium**, or *Chlordiazepoxide*) 83
Clopress (**Anafranil**, or *Clomipramine*) 43
Clorazepate (**Tranxene**) 83
Clorazepate dipotassium (**Tranxene**, or *Clorazepate*) 83
Clorazepic acid (**Tranxene**, or *Clorazepate*) 83
Clordiazepossido (**Librium**, or *Chlordiazepoxide*) 83
Clostedal (**Tegretol**, or *Carbamazepine*) 77
Cloxazepine (**Loxitane**, or *Loxapine*) 101
Clozapin (**Clozaril**, or *Clozapine*) 108
Clozapine (**Clozaril**) 108
Clozaril (*Clozapine*) 108
Combid (**Compazine**, or *Prochlorperazine*) 100
Compazine (*Prochlorperazine*) 100
Compro (**Compazine**, or *Prochlorperazine*) 100
Concerta (**Ritalin**, or *Methylphenidate*) 63
Concordin (**Surmontil**, or *Trimipramine*) 43
Concordine (**Surmontil**, or *Trimipramine*) 43
Condition (**Valium**, or *Diazepam*) 83
Constan (**Xanax**, or *Alprazolam*) 83
Constimol (**Cylert**, or *Pemoline*) 63
Contemnol (**Lithobid**, or *Lithium Carbonate*) 73
Contol (**Librium**, or *Chlordiazepoxide*) 83
Contomin (**Thorazine**, or *Chlorpromazine*) 100
Control (**Librium**, or *Chlordiazepoxide*) 83
Convulex (**Depakote**, or *Divalproex*) 75
Convulex Syrup (**Depacon**, or *Sodium Valproate*) 75

Convuline (**Tegretol**, or *Carbamazepine*) 77
Coolspan (**Dolmatil**, or *Sulpiride*) 108
CPT (**Truxal**, or *Chlorprothixene*) 101
CPX (**Truxal**, or *Chlorprothixene*) 101
CPZ (**Thorazine**, or *Chlorpromazine*) 100
Curatin (**Sinequan**, or *Doxepin*) 43
Cylert (*Pemoline*) 63
Cylert Chewable (**Cylert**, or *Pemoline*) 63
Cymbalta (*Duloxetine*) 50
Cypoheptadine (**Periactin**, or *Cyproheptadine*) 122
Cyprenil (**Eldepryl**, or *Selegiline (oral)*) 37
Cyproheptadine (**Periactin**) 122
Cyproheptadiene (**Periactin**, or *Cyproheptadine*) 122
D 65MT (**Xanax**, or *Alprazolam*) 83
Dalcipran (*Milnacipran*) 50
Damilan (**Elavil**, or *Amitriptyline*) 43
Damilen (**Elavil**, or *Amitriptyline*) 43
Damitriptyline (**Elavil**, or *Amitriptyline*) 43
Dantromin (**Cylert**, or *Pemoline*) 63
DAP (**Valium**, or *Diazepam*) 83
Darleton (**Dolmatil**, or *Sulpiride*) 108
Dayto Himbin (**Yocon**, or *Yohimbine*) 116
Dea No. 1680 (**Provigil**, or *Modafinil*) 63
Decacil (**Librium**, or *Chlordiazepoxide*) 83
Decentan (**Trilafon**, or *Perphenazine*) 100
Declomipramine (**Tofranil**, or *Imipramine*) 43
Defanyl (**Asendin**, or *Amoxapine*) 43
Degranol (**Tegretol**, or *Carbamazepine*) 77
Dehidrobenzperidol (**Inapsine**, or *Droperidol*) 102
Dehydrobenzperidol (**Inapsine**, or *Droperidol*) 102
Deidrobenzperidolo (**Inapsine**, or *Droperidol*) 102
Delepsine (**Depakene**, or *Valproic Acid*) 75
Delormetazepam (**Ativan**, or *Lorazepam*) 83
Deltamin (**Cylert**, or *Pemoline*) 63
Deltamine (**Cylert**, or *Pemoline*) 63
Demethyl-Amitryptyline (**Pamelor**, or *Nortriptyline*) 43
Demethylamitriptylene (**Pamelor**, or *Nortriptyline*) 43
Demethylamitriptyline (**Pamelor**, or *Nortriptyline*) 43
Demethylamitryptyline (**Pamelor**, or *Nortriptyline*) 43
Demethylimipramine (**Norpramin**, or *Desipramine*) 43
Demolox (**Asendin**, or *Amoxapine*) 43
Deoxy-Norephedrine (**Dexedrine**, or *Dextroamphetamine*) 63
Depacon (*Sodium Valproate*) 75

Depakene (*Valproic Acid*) 75
Depakin (**Depacon**, or *Sodium Valproate*) 75
Depakine (**Depakote**, or *Divalproex*) 75
Depakine Depakote (**Depacon**, or *Sodium Valproate*) 75
Depakote (*Divalproex*) 75
Depalept (**Depacon**, or *Sodium Valproate*) 75
Depalept Chrono (**Depacon**, or *Sodium Valproate*) 75
Depixol (*Flupenthixol*) 101
Deprax (**Desyrel**, or *Trazodone*) 49
Deprenyl (**Eldepryl**, or *Selegiline (oral)*) 37
Deprex (**Prozac**, or *Fluoxetine*) 47
Deprilept (**Ludiomil**, or *Maprotiline*) 43
Deproic (**Depakene**, or *Valproic Acid*) 75
Depromel (**Luvox**, or *Fluvoxamine*) 47
Deproxin (**Prozac**, or *Fluoxetine*) 47
Deroxat (**Paxil**, or *Paroxetine*) 47
Desidox (**Sinequan**, or *Doxepin*) 43
Desimipramine (**Norpramin**, or *Desipramine*) 43
Desimpramine (**Norpramin**, or *Desipramine*) 43
Desipramine (**Norpramin**) 43
Desipramin (**Norpramin**, or *Desipramine*) 43
Desirel (**Desyrel**, or *Trazodone*) 49
Desitriptilina (**Pamelor**, or *Nortriptyline*) 43
Desmenat (**Dolmatil**, or *Sulpiride*) 108
Desmethylamitriptyline (**Pamelor**, or *Nortriptyline*) 43
Desmethylimipramine (**Norpramin**, or *Desipramine*) 43
Desoxyn (**Dexedrine**, or *Dextroamphetamine*) 63
(+/-)-Desoxynorephedrine (**Dexedrine**, or *Dextroamphetamine*) 63
Desyrel (*Trazodone*) 49
Dexampex (**Dexedrine**, or *Dextroamphetamine*) 63
Dexedrine (*Dextroamphetamine*) 63
Dextroamphetamine (**Dexedrine**) 63
Dextroamphetamine Sulfate (**Dexedrine**, or *Dextroamphetamine*) 63
Dextrostat (**Dexedrine**, or *Dextroamphetamine*) 63
Dezipramine (**Norpramin**, or *Desipramine*) 43
DHBP (**Inapsine**, or *Droperidol*) 102
Di-n-propylacetic acid (**Depakene**, or *Valproic Acid*) 75
Di-n-propylessigsaure (**Depakene**, or *Valproic Acid*) 75
Diacepan (**Valium**, or *Diazepam*) 83
Dialag (**Valium**, or *Diazepam*) 83
Dialar (**Valium**, or *Diazepam*) 83
Diapam (**Valium**, or *Diazepam*) 83
Diastat (**Valium**, or *Diazepam*) 83

Diazemuls (**Valium**, or *Diazepam*) 83
Diazemulus (**Valium**, or *Diazepam*) 83
Diazepam (**Valium**) 83
Diazepam Intensol (**Valium**, or *Diazepam*) 83
Diazepan (**Valium**, or *Diazepam*) 83
Diazetard (**Valium**, or *Diazepam*) 83
Dibenzacepin (**Loxitane**, or *Loxapine*) 101
Dibenzoazepine (**Loxitane**, or *Loxapine*) 101
Dibenzosuberonone/Cyproheptadine (**Periactin**, or *Cyproheptadine*) 122
Dienpax (**Valium**, or *Diazepam*) 83
Dihidrobenzperidol (**Inapsine**, or *Droperidol*) 102
Dimethylimipramine (**Norpramin**, or *Desipramine*) 43
Dimipressin (**Tofranil**, or *Imipramine*) 43
Dipam (**Valium**, or *Diazepam*) 83
Dipezona (**Valium**, or *Diazepam*) 83
Dipropylacetic acid (**Depakote**, or *Divalproex*) 75
Directim (**Survector**, or *Amineptine*) 56
Divalproex (**Depakote**) 75
Divalproex sodium (**Depakote**, or *Divalproex*) 75
Dizac (**Valium**, or *Diazepam*) 83
Dl-1-Phenyl-2-aminopropane (**Dexedrine**, or *Dextroamphetamine*) 63
DL-alpha-Methylphenethylamine (**Dexedrine**, or *Dextroamphetamine*) 63
Dl-Amphetamine (**Dexedrine**, or *Dextroamphetamine*) 63
Dl-Benzedrine (**Dexedrine**, or *Dextroamphetamine*) 63
Dl-Tranylcypromine (**Parnate**, or *Tranylcypromine*) 39
DMI (**Norpramin**, or *Desipramine*) 43
Dobren (**Dolmatil**, or *Sulpiride*) 108
Dogmatil (**Dolmatil**, or *Sulpiride*) 108
Dogmatyl (**Dolmatil**, or *Sulpiride*) 108
Dolmatil (*Sulpiride*) 108
Dom-Valproic (**Depakene**, or *Valproic Acid*) 75
Domalium (**Valium**, or *Diazepam*) 83
Domical (**Elavil**, or *Amitriptyline*) 43
Domperidone (**Cymbalta**, or *Duloxetine*) 50
Doneurin (**Sinequan**, or *Doxepin*) 43
Dostinex (*Cabergoline*) 59
Dosulepin (**Prothiaden**, or *Dothiepin*) 43
Dosulepine (**Prothiaden**, or *Dothiepin*) 43
Dothapax (**Prothiaden**, or *Dothiepin*) 43
Dothep (**Prothiaden**, or *Dothiepin*) 43
Dothiepin (**Prothiaden**) 43
Doxal (**Sinequan**, or *Doxepin*) 43
Doxedyn (**Sinequan**, or *Doxepin*) 43

Eldepryl (*Selegiline (oral)*) 37

Elenium (**Librium**, or *Chlordiazepoxide*) 83

Elinol (**Prolixin Injection**, or *Fluphenazine Decanoate*) 100

Elmarin (**Sparine**, or *Promazine*) 100

Elvetium (**Depakote**, or *Divalproex*) 75

Emelent (**Compazine**, or *Prochlorperazine*) 100

Emergil (**Depixol**, or *Flupenthixol*) 101

Emesinal (**Trilafon**, or *Perphenazine*) 100

Emetiral (**Compazine**, or *Prochlorperazine*) 100

Emitrip (**Elavil**, or *Amitriptyline*) 43

Emotival (**Ativan**, or *Lorazepam*) 83

Emsam (*Selegiline (patch)*) 37

Endantadine (**Symmetrel**, or *Amantadine*) 59

Endep (**Elavil**, or *Amitriptyline*) 43

Endolin (**Cylert**, or *Pemoline*) 63

Enerzer (**Marplan**, or *Isocarboxazid*) 39

Enimon (**Dolmatil**, or *Sulpiride*) 108

Enovil (**Elavil**, or *Amitriptyline*) 43

Epiject (**Depakene**, or *Valproic Acid*) 75

Epilam (**Depacon**, or *Sodium Valproate*) 75

Epileptol (**Tegretol**, or *Carbamazepine*) 77

Epileptol CR (**Tegretol**, or *Carbamazepine*) 77

Epilex (**Depacon**, or *Sodium Valproate*) 75

Epilim (**Depakote**, or *Divalproex*) 75

Epilim Chrono (**Depacon**, or *Sodium Valproate*) 75

Epitol (**Tegretol**, or *Carbamazepine*) 77

Epival (**Depakote**, or *Divalproex*) 75

Eposal Retard (**Tegretol**, or *Carbamazepine*) 77

Equetro (**Tegretol**, or *Carbamazepine*) 77

Equilid (**Dolmatil**, or *Sulpiride*) 108

Ergenyl (**Depakote**, or *Divalproex*) 75

Eridan (**Valium**, or *Diazepam*) 83

Erocap (**Prozac**, or *Fluoxetine*) 47

Escitalopram (**Lexapro**) 47

Escitalopram Oxalate (**Lexapro**, or *Escitalopram*) 47

Eskalith (**Lithobid**, or *Lithium Carbonate*) 73

Eskalith-Cr (**Lithobid**, or *Lithium Carbonate*) 73

Eskatrol (**Compazine**, or *Prochlorperazine*) 100

Eskazine (**Stelazine**, or *Trifluoperazine*) 100

Eskazinyl (**Stelazine**, or *Trifluoperazine*) 100

Esmind (**Sparine**, or *Promazine*) 100

Espa-lepsin (**Tegretol**, or *Carbamazepine*) 77

Esparin (**Sparine**, or *Promazine*) 100

Fluanxol Depot (**Depixol**, or *Flupenthixol*) 101

Fluctin (**Prozac**, or *Fluoxetine*) 47

Fluctine (**Prozac**, or *Fluoxetine*) 47

Fludac (**Prozac**, or *Fluoxetine*) 47

Flufran (**Prozac**, or *Fluoxetine*) 47

Flunil (**Prozac**, or *Fluoxetine*) 47

Fluoperazine (**Stelazine**, or *Trifluoperazine*) 100

Fluorfenazine (**Prolixin Injection**, or *Fluphenazine Decanoate*) 100

Fluorophenazine (**Prolixin Injection**, or *Fluphenazine Decanoate*) 100

Fluorphenazine (**Prolixin Injection**, or *Fluphenazine Decanoate*) 100

Fluoxac (**Prozac**, or *Fluoxetine*) 47

Fluoxeren (**Prozac**, or *Fluoxetine*) 47

Fluoxetina (**Prozac**, or *Fluoxetine*) 47

Fluoxetine (**Prozac**) 47

Fluoxetine + Olanzapine (**Symbyax**) 47

Fluoxetinum (**Prozac**, or *Fluoxetine*) 47

Fluoxil (**Prozac**, or *Fluoxetine*) 47

Flupenthixol (**Depixol**) 101

Flupenthixole (**Depixol**, or *Flupenthixol*) 101

Flupentixol (**Depixol**, or *Flupenthixol*) 101

Fluphenazine Decanoate (**Prolixin Injection**) 100

Fluphenazine (**Trilafon**, or *Perphenazine*) 100

Flurentixol (**Depixol**, or *Flupenthixol*) 101

Flutin (**Prozac**, or *Fluoxetine*) 47

Flutine (**Prozac**, or *Fluoxetine*) 47

Fluval (**Prozac**, or *Fluoxetine*) 47

Fluvoxamine (**Luvox**) 47

Fluvoxamina (**Luvox**, or *Fluvoxamine*) 47

Fluvoxamine maleate (**Luvox**, or *Fluvoxamine*) 47

Fluvoxaminum (**Luvox**, or *Fluvoxamine*) 47

Fluxanxol (**Depixol**, or *Flupenthixol*) 101

Fluxil (**Prozac**, or *Fluoxetine*) 47

Focalin (**Ritalin**, or *Methylphenidate*) 63

Focalin XR (**Ritalin**, or *Methylphenidate*) 63

Fontex (**Prozac**, or *Fluoxetine*) 47

Foxalepsin (**Tegretol**, or *Carbamazepine*) 77

Foxalepsin Retard (**Tegretol**, or *Carbamazepine*) 77

Foxetin (**Prozac**, or *Fluoxetine*) 47

Fraction (**Sparine**, or *Promazine*) 100

Freudal (**Valium**, or *Diazepam*) 83

Frontal (**Xanax**, or *Alprazolam*) 83

Frustan (**Valium**, or *Diazepam*) 83

Furfuryl Acetate (**Mirapex**, or *Pramipexole*) 59

Hyton asa (**Cylert**, or *Pemoline*) 63
Iaractan (**Truxal**, or *Chlorprothixene*) 101
ICOS 351 (**Cialis**, or *Tadalafil*) 114
Ictho-Himbin (**Yocon**, or *Yohimbine*) 116
Idalprem (**Ativan**, or *Lorazepam*) 83
Ifibrium (**Librium**, or *Chlordiazepoxide*) 83
Iktorivil (**Klonopin**, or *Clonazepam*) 83
IM (**Tofranil**, or *Imipramine*) 43
Imavate (**Tofranil**, or *Imipramine*) 43
Imidobenzyle (**Tofranil**, or *Imipramine*) 43
Imipramine (**Tofranil**) 43
Imipramina (**Tofranil**, or *Imipramine*) 43
Imiprin (**Tofranil**, or *Imipramine*) 43
Imizin (**Tofranil**, or *Imipramine*) 43
Imizine (**Tofranil**, or *Imipramine*) 43
Imizinum (**Tofranil**, or *Imipramine*) 43
Impramine (**Tofranil**, or *Imipramine*) 43
Impril (**Tofranil**, or *Imipramine*) 43
Inappin (**Inapsine**, or *Droperidol*) 102
Inapsin (**Inapsine**, or *Droperidol*) 102
Inapsine (*Droperidol*) 102
Innovan (**Inapsine**, or *Droperidol*) 102
Innovar (**Inapsine**, or *Droperidol*) 102
Innovar-Vet (**Inapsine**, or *Droperidol*) 102
Inopsin (**Inapsine**, or *Droperidol*) 102
Inoval (**Inapsine**, or *Droperidol*) 102
Intalpram (**Tofranil**, or *Imipramine*) 43
Intensol (**Xanax**, or *Alprazolam*) 83
Invega (*Paliperidone*) 108
Iprox (**Clozaril**, or *Clozapine*) 108
Iramil (**Tofranil**, or *Imipramine*) 43
Irmin (**Tofranil**, or *Imipramine*) 43
Isnamide (**Dolmatil**, or *Sulpiride*) 108
Isoamycin (**Dexedrine**, or *Dextroamphetamine*) 63
Isoamyne (**Dexedrine**, or *Dextroamphetamine*) 63
Isocarboxazid (**Marplan**) 39
Isocarbonazid (**Marplan**, or *Isocarboxazid*) 39
Isocarbossazide (**Marplan**, or *Isocarboxazid*) 39
Isocarboxazida (**Marplan**, or *Isocarboxazid*) 39
Isocarboxazide (**Marplan**, or *Isocarboxazid*) 39
Isocarboxazidum (**Marplan**, or *Isocarboxazid*) 39
Isocarboxyzid (**Marplan**, or *Isocarboxazid*) 39
Isomyn (**Dexedrine**, or *Dextroamphetamine*) 63

Lepotex (**Clozaril**, or *Clozapine*) 108
Leptanal (**Inapsine**, or *Droperidol*) 102
Leptilan (**Depacon**, or *Sodium Valproate*) 75
Leptofen (**Inapsine**, or *Droperidol*) 102
Lesotal (**Eldepryl**, or *Selegiline (oral)*) 37
Levate (**Elavil**, or *Amitriptyline*) 43
Levitra (*Vardenafil*) 114
Levium (**Valium**, or *Diazepam*) 83
Levobren (**Dolmatil**, or *Sulpiride*) 108
Levopraid (**Dolmatil**, or *Sulpiride*) 108
Levosulpirida (**Dolmatil**, or *Sulpiride*) 108
Levosulpiride (**Dolmatil**, or *Sulpiride*) 108
Levosulpiridum (**Dolmatil**, or *Sulpiride*) 108
Lexapro (*Escitalopram*) 47
Lexin (**Tegretol**, or *Carbamazepine*) 77
Liberetas (**Valium**, or *Diazepam*) 83
Librax (**Librium**, or *Chlordiazepoxide*) 83
Librelease (**Librium**, or *Chlordiazepoxide*) 83
Librinin (**Librium**, or *Chlordiazepoxide*) 83
Libritabs (**Librium**, or *Chlordiazepoxide*) 83
Librium (*Chlordiazepoxide*) 83
Licab (**Lithobid**, or *Lithium Carbonate*) 73
Licarb (**Lithobid**, or *Lithium Carbonate*) 73
Licarbium (**Lithobid**, or *Lithium Carbonate*) 73
Lidanar (**Serentil**, or *Mesoridazine*) 100
Lidanil (**Serentil**, or *Mesoridazine*) 100
Lidin (**Lithobid**, or *Lithium Carbonate*) 73
Lidone (**Moban**, or *Molindone*) 101
Limas (**Lithobid**, or *Lithium Carbonate*) 73
Limbitrol (**Librium**, or *Chlordiazepoxide*) 83
Limbitrol Ds (**Librium**, or *Chlordiazepoxide*) 83
Linton (**Haldol**, or *Haloperidol*) 101
Liranol (**Sparine**, or *Promazine*) 100
Lisdexamfetamine (**Vyvanse**) 63
Liskonum (**Lithobid**, or *Lithium Carbonate*) 73
Lisopiride (**Dolmatil**, or *Sulpiride*) 108
Litarex (**Lithobid**, or *Lithium Carbonate*) 73
Lithane (**Lithobid**, or *Lithium Carbonate*) 73
Litheum 300 (**Lithobid**, or *Lithium Carbonate*) 73
Lithicarb (**Lithobid**, or *Lithium Carbonate*) 73
Lithionate (**Lithobid**, or *Lithium Carbonate*) 73
Lithium Carbonate (**Lithobid**) 73
Lithium Citrate (**Priadel**) 73

Lithizine (**Lithobid**, or *Lithium Carbonate*) 73

Lithobid (*Lithium Carbonate*) 73

Lithocap (**Lithobid**, or *Lithium Carbonate*) 73

Lithonate (**Lithobid**, or *Lithium Carbonate*) 73

Lithotabs (**Lithobid**, or *Lithium Carbonate*) 73

Litilent (**Lithobid**, or *Lithium Carbonate*) 73

Litocarb (**Lithobid**, or *Lithium Carbonate*) 73

Lorabenz (**Ativan**, or *Lorazepam*) 83

Lorax (**Ativan**, or *Lorazepam*) 83

Loraz (**Ativan**, or *Lorazepam*) 83

Lorazepam (**Ativan**) 83

Lorazepam Intensol (**Ativan**, or *Lorazepam*) 83

(+/-)-Lorazepam (**Ativan**, or *Lorazepam*) 83

Lorien (**Prozac**, or *Fluoxetine*) 47

Lorsilan (**Ativan**, or *Lorazepam*) 83

Lossapina (**Loxitane**, or *Loxapine*) 101

Lovan (**Prozac**, or *Fluoxetine*) 47

Loxapac (**Loxitane**, or *Loxapine*) 101

Loxapin (**Loxitane**, or *Loxapine*) 101

Loxapina (**Loxitane**, or *Loxapine*) 101

Loxapine (**Loxitane**) 101

Loxapine Succinate (**Loxitane**, or *Loxapine*) 101

Loxapinum (**Loxitane**, or *Loxapine*) 101

Loxepine (**Loxitane**, or *Loxapine*) 101

Loxitane (*Loxapine*) 101

Loxitane C (**Loxitane**, or *Loxapine*) 101

Loxitane Im (**Loxitane**, or *Loxapine*) 101

Lucelan (**BuSpar**, or *Buspirone*) 119

Ludiomil (*Maprotiline*) 43

Lumbeck (**Pamelor**, or *Nortriptyline*) 43

Lumin (**Paxil**, or *Paroxetine*) 47

Lustral (**Zoloft**, or *Sertraline*) 47

Luvox (*Fluvoxamine*) 47

Luvoxe (**Luvox**, or *Fluvoxamine*) 47

Lygen (**Librium**, or *Chlordiazepoxide*) 83

M-Methoxy-a-methylphenethylamine (**Dexedrine**, or *Dextroamphetamine*) 63

M-Methoxyamphetamine (**Dexedrine**, or *Dextroamphetamine*) 63

Macrepan (**Tegretol**, or *Carbamazepine*) 77

Mallorol (**Mellaril**, or *Thioridazine*) 100

Malloryl (**Mellaril**, or *Thioridazine*) 100

Maludil (**Ludiomil**, or *Maprotiline*) 43

Mandrozep (**Valium**, or *Diazepam*) 83

Manegan (**Desyrel**, or *Trazodone*) 49

Maneon (**Survector**, or *Amineptine*) 56
Manerix (*Moclobemide*) 35
Maniprex (**Lithobid**, or *Lithium Carbonate*) 73
Mantadine (**Symmetrel**, or *Amantadine*) 59
Maprotiline (**Ludiomil**) 43
Maprotilina (**Ludiomil**, or *Maprotiline*) 43
Maprotilinum (**Ludiomil**, or *Maprotiline*) 43
Maprotylina (**Ludiomil**, or *Maprotiline*) 43
Maraplan (**Marplan**, or *Isocarboxazid*) 39
Margrilan (**Prozac**, or *Fluoxetine*) 47
Mariastel (**Dolmatil**, or *Sulpiride*) 108
Marplan (*Isocarboxazid*) 39
Marplon (**Marplan**, or *Isocarboxazid*) 39
Maveral (**Luvox**, or *Fluvoxamine*) 47
Maximed (**Surmontil**, or *Trimipramine*) 43
Mazetol (**Tegretol**, or *Carbamazepine*) 77
McN-JR 749 (**Inapsine**, or *Droperidol*) 102
Mechotane (**Urecholine**, or *Bethanechol*) 123
Mechothane (**Urecholine**, or *Bethanechol*) 123
Mecodrin (**Dexedrine**, or *Dextroamphetamine*) 63
Mecothane (**Urecholine**, or *Bethanechol*) 123
Med Valproic (**Depakene**, or *Valproic Acid*) 75
Megaphen (**Sparine**, or *Promazine*) 100
Meleril (**Mellaril**, or *Thioridazine*) 100
Melipramin (**Tofranil**, or *Imipramine*) 43
Melipramine (**Tofranil**, or *Imipramine*) 43
Mellaril (*Thioridazine*) 100
Mellaril-S (**Mellaril**, or *Thioridazine*) 100
Mellarit (**Mellaril**, or *Thioridazine*) 100
Mellerets (**Mellaril**, or *Thioridazine*) 100
Mellerette (**Mellaril**, or *Thioridazine*) 100
Melleretten (**Mellaril**, or *Thioridazine*) 100
Melleril (**Mellaril**, or *Thioridazine*) 100
Melodil (**Ludiomil**, or *Maprotiline*) 43
Menfazona (**Serzone**, or *Nefazodone*) 49
Menrium (**Librium**, or *Chlordiazepoxide*) 83
Mepirzepine (**Remeron**, or *Mirtazapine*) 54
Meresa (**Dolmatil**, or *Sulpiride*) 108
Meridil (**Ritalin**, or *Methylphenidate*) 63
Mesoridazine (**Serentil**) 100
Mesural (**Librium**, or *Chlordiazepoxide*) 83
Metadate (**Ritalin**, or *Methylphenidate*) 63
Metadate CD (**Ritalin**, or *Methylphenidate*) 63

Mirtazepine (**Remeron**, or *Mirtazapine*) 54
Misulvan (**Dolmatil**, or *Sulpiride*) 108
Mixidol (**Haldol**, or *Haloperidol*) 101
Moban (*Molindone*) 101
Moclaime (**Manerix**, or *Moclobemide*) 35
Moclamide (**Manerix**, or *Moclobemide*) 35
Moclamine (**Manerix**, or *Moclobemide*) 35
Moclobemide (**Manerix**) 35
Moclobemid (**Manerix**, or *Moclobemide*) 35
Moclobemida (**Manerix**, or *Moclobemide*) 35
Moclobemidum (**Manerix**, or *Moclobemide*) 35
Modafinil (**Provigil**) 63
Modafinilo (**Provigil**, or *Modafinil*) 63
Modafinilum (**Provigil**, or *Modafinil*) 63
Modalina (**Stelazine**, or *Trifluoperazine*) 100
Modecate (**Prolixin Injection**, or *Fluphenazine Decanoate*) 100
Moderateafinil (**Provigil**, or *Modafinil*) 63
Modiodal (**Provigil**, or *Modafinil*) 63
Modipran (**Prozac**, or *Fluoxetine*) 47
Moditen (**Prolixin Injection**, or *Fluphenazine Decanoate*) 100
Moditen Enanthate (**Prolixin Injection**, or *Fluphenazine Decanoate*) 100
Moditen Hcl (**Prolixin Injection**, or *Fluphenazine Decanoate*) 100
Modobemde (**Manerix**, or *Moclobemide*) 35
Molindone (**Moban**) 101
Molipaxin (**Desyrel**, or *Trazodone*) 49
Monochlorimipramine (**Anafranil**, or *Clomipramine*) 43
Monodemethylimipramine (**Norpramin**, or *Desipramine*) 43
Monofen (**Nardil**, or *Phenelzine*) 39
Morosan (**Valium**, or *Diazepam*) 83
Movergan (**Eldepryl**, or *Selegiline (oral)*) 37
Moxadil (**Asendin**, or *Amoxapine*) 43
Multum (**Librium**, or *Chlordiazepoxide*) 83
Muse (*Alprostadil*) 114
Myamin (**Cylert**, or *Pemoline*) 63
Mylproin (**Depakote**, or *Divalproex*) 75
Myocholine (**Urecholine**, or *Bethanechol*) 123
Myotonachol (**Urecholine**, or *Bethanechol*) 123
Myotonine Chloride (**Urecholine**, or *Bethanechol*) 123
Myproic Acid (**Depakene**, or *Valproic Acid*) 75
N-dipropylacetic acid (**Depakote**, or *Divalproex*) 75
N-DPA (**Depakote**, or *Divalproex*) 75
Napoton (**Librium**, or *Chlordiazepoxide*) 83
Napton (**Librium**, or *Chlordiazepoxide*) 83

Nortriptyline (**Pamelor**) 43
Nortryptiline (**Pamelor**, or *Nortriptyline*) 43
Norzepine (**Pamelor**, or *Nortriptyline*) 43
Notair (**Cylert**, or *Pemoline*) 63
Novamin (**Compazine**, or *Prochlorperazine*) 100
Novazam (**Valium**, or *Diazepam*) 83
Novo-Carbamaz (**Tegretol**, or *Carbamazepine*) 77
Novo-Chlorpromazine (**Thorazine**, or *Chlorpromazine*) 100
Novo-Dipam (**Valium**, or *Diazepam*) 83
Novo-Doxepin (**Sinequan**, or *Doxepin*) 43
Novo-Gabapentin (**Neurontin**, or *Gabapentin*) 79
Novo-Peridol (**Haldol**, or *Haloperidol*) 101
Novo-Poxide (**Librium**, or *Chlordiazepoxide*) 83
Novo-Selegiline (**Eldepryl**, or *Selegiline (oral)*) 37
Novo-Trifluzine (**Stelazine**, or *Trifluoperazine*) 100
Novo-Tripramine (**Vivactil**, or *Protriptyline*) 43
Novo-Valproic (**Depakene**, or *Valproic Acid*) 75
Novomazina (**Sparine**, or *Promazine*) 100
Novopramine (**Tofranil**, or *Imipramine*) 43
Novoridazine (**Mellaril**, or *Thioridazine*) 100
Novoseven (**Depakote**, or *Divalproex*) 75
Novotriptyn (**Elavil**, or *Amitriptyline*) 43
Novydrine (**Dexedrine**, or *Dextroamphetamine*) 63
NPL 1 (**Cylert**, or *Pemoline*) 63
Nu-Carbamazepine (**Tegretol**, or *Carbamazepine*) 77
Nu-Selegiline (**Eldepryl**, or *Selegiline (oral)*) 37
Nu-Valproic (**Depakene**, or *Valproic Acid*) 75
Nufarol (**Dolmatil**, or *Sulpiride*) 108
O-Chlorooxazepam (**Ativan**, or *Lorazepam*) 83
O-Chloroxazepam (**Ativan**, or *Lorazepam*) 83
Okodon (**Cylert**, or *Pemoline*) 63
Oktedrin (**Dexedrine**, or *Dextroamphetamine*) 63
Olansek (**Zyprexa**, or *Olanzapine*) 108
Olanzapine (**Zyprexa**) 108
Olsalazine (**Remeron**, or *Mirtazapine*) 54
Omca (**Prolixin Injection**, or *Fluphenazine Decanoate*) 100
Omiryl (**Dolmatil**, or *Sulpiride*) 108
Omperan (**Dolmatil**, or *Sulpiride*) 108
OPC 31 (**Abilify**, or *Aripiprazole*) 108
Opiran (**Orap**, or *Pimozide*) 102
Optimax (*L-Tryptophan*) 28
Orap (*Pimozide*) 102
Orfil (**Depacon**, or *Sodium Valproate*) 75

Orfiril (**Depacon**, or *Sodium Valproate*) 75
Orfiril Retard (**Depacon**, or *Sodium Valproate*) 75
Orsanil (**Mellaril**, or *Thioridazine*) 100
Ortedrine (**Dexedrine**, or *Dextroamphetamine*) 63
Oxaprozin (**Trileptal**, or *Oxcarbazepine*) 77
Oxaprozine (**Trileptal**, or *Oxcarbazepine*) 77
Oxcarbazepine (**Trileptal**) 77
Oxcarbamazepine (**Trileptal**, or *Oxcarbazepine*) 77
Oxedep (**Prozac**, or *Fluoxetine*) 47
Oxilapine (**Loxitane**, or *Loxapine*) 101
Ozoderpin (**Dolmatil**, or *Sulpiride*) 108
Paceum (**Valium**, or *Diazepam*) 83
Pacinol (**Prolixin Injection**, or *Fluphenazine Decanoate*) 100
Pacitran (**Valium**, or *Diazepam*) 83
Paliperidone (**Invega**) 108
Pamelor (*Nortriptyline*) 43
Panitol (**Tegretol**, or *Carbamazepine*) 77
Paranten (**Valium**, or *Diazepam*) 83
Paredrine (**Dexedrine**, or *Dextroamphetamine*) 63
Parlodel (*Bromocriptine*) 59
Parmodalin (**Parnate**, or *Tranylcypromine*) 39
Parnate (*Tranylcypromine*) 39
Paroxetina (**Paxil**, or *Paroxetine*) 47
Paroxetine (**Paxil**) 47
Paroxetinum (**Paxil**, or *Paroxetine*) 47
Pasotomin (**Compazine**, or *Prochlorperazine*) 100
Pasuma (**Yocon**, or *Yohimbine*) 116
Paxate (**Valium**, or *Diazepam*) 83
Paxel (**Valium**, or *Diazepam*) 83
Paxil (*Paroxetine*) 47
Paxil Cr (**Paxil**, or *Paroxetine*) 47
Paxyl (**Truxal**, or *Chlorprothixene*) 101
Pekuces (**Haldol**, or *Haloperidol*) 101
Peluces (**Haldol**, or *Haloperidol*) 101
Pemolin (**Cylert**, or *Pemoline*) 63
Pemolina (**Cylert**, or *Pemoline*) 63
Pemoline (**Cylert**) 63
Penta-Valproic (**Depakene**, or *Valproic Acid*) 75
Pentofran (**Norpramin**, or *Desipramine*) 43
Percomon (**Dexedrine**, or *Dextroamphetamine*) 63
Perfenazina (**Trilafon**, or *Perphenazine*) 100
Perfenazine (**Trilafon**, or *Perphenazine*) 100
Pergolida (**Permax**, or *Pergolide*) 59

Pergolide (**Permax**) 59
Pergolide Mesylate (**Permax**, or *Pergolide*) 59
Pergolide Methanesulfonate (**Permax**, or *Pergolide*) 59
Pergolidum (**Permax**, or *Pergolide*) 59
Periactin (*Cyproheptadine*) 122
Periactine (**Periactin**, or *Cyproheptadine*) 122
Periactinol (**Periactin**, or *Cyproheptadine*) 122
Peridol (**Haldol**, or *Haloperidol*) 101
Peritol (**Periactin**, or *Cyproheptadine*) 122
Permax (*Pergolide*) 59
Permitil (**Prolixin Injection**, or *Fluphenazine Decanoate*) 100
Pernox (**Haldol**, or *Haloperidol*) 101
Perphenazine (**Trilafon**) 100
Perphenan (**Trilafon**, or *Perphenazine*) 100
Perphenazin (**Trilafon**, or *Perphenazine*) 100
Perphenazine (**Prolixin Injection**, or *Fluphenazine Decanoate*) 100
Pertofran (**Norpramin**, or *Desipramine*) 43
Pertofrane (**Norpramin**, or *Desipramine*) 43
Pertofrin (**Norpramin**, or *Desipramine*) 43
Pertrofane (**Norpramin**, or *Desipramine*) 43
Petilin (**Depacon**, or *Sodium Valproate*) 75
Pexeva (**Paxil**, or *Paroxetine*) 47
PGE1 (**Muse**, or *Alprostadil*) 114
Phanate (**Lithobid**, or *Lithium Carbonate*) 73
Pharmaceutical (**Valium**, or *Diazepam*) 83
Phasal (**Lithobid**, or *Lithium Carbonate*) 73
Phenalone (**Cylert**, or *Pemoline*) 63
Phenalzine (**Nardil**, or *Phenelzine*) 39
Phenamine (**Dexedrine**, or *Dextroamphetamine*) 63
Phenedrine (**Dexedrine**, or *Dextroamphetamine*) 63
Phenelezine (**Nardil**, or *Phenelzine*) 39
Phenelzine (**Nardil**) 39
Phenelzinum (**Nardil**, or *Phenelzine*) 39
Phenethylhydrazine (**Nardil**, or *Phenelzine*) 39
Phenidylate (**Ritalin**, or *Methylphenidate*) 63
Phenilone (**Cylert**, or *Pemoline*) 63
Pheniminooxazolidinone (**Cylert**, or *Pemoline*) 63
Phenothiazine (**Sparine**, or *Promazine*) 100
Phenoxazole (**Cylert**, or *Pemoline*) 63
1-Phenyl-2-aminopropane (**Dexedrine**, or *Dextroamphetamine*) 63
Phenylethyl hydrazine-HCl (**Nardil**, or *Phenelzine*) 39
Phenylethylhydrazine (**Nardil**, or *Phenelzine*) 39
Phenylisohydantoin (**Cylert**, or *Pemoline*) 63

Primozida (**Orap**, or *Pimozide*) 102
Prink (**Muse**, or *Alprostadil*) 114
Prizma (**Prozac**, or *Fluoxetine*) 47
Pro Dorm (**Ativan**, or *Lorazepam*) 83
Pro-Pam (**Valium**, or *Diazepam*) 83
Proavil (**Trilafon**, or *Perphenazine*) 100
Prochlorperazine (**Compazine**) 100
Prochloroperazine (**Compazine**, or *Prochlorperazine*) 100
Prochlorpemazine (**Compazine**, or *Prochlorperazine*) 100
Prochlorperazin (**Compazine**, or *Prochlorperazine*) 100
Prochlorperazine edisylate (**Compazine**, or *Prochlorperazine*) 100
Prochlorperazine maleate (**Compazine**, or *Prochlorperazine*) 100
Prochlorpromazine (**Compazine**, or *Prochlorperazine*) 100
Procloperazine (**Compazine**, or *Prochlorperazine*) 100
Proclorperazine (**Compazine**, or *Prochlorperazine*) 100
Prodep (**Prozac**, or *Fluoxetine*) 47
Profamina (**Dexedrine**, or *Dextroamphetamine*) 63
Proheptadiene (**Elavil**, or *Amitriptyline*) 43
Prolixin Decanoate (**Prolixin Injection**, or *Fluphenazine Decanoate*) 100
Prolixin Enanthate (**Prolixin Injection**, or *Fluphenazine Decanoate*) 100
Prolixin Injection (*Fluphenazine Decanoate*) 100
Prolixine (**Prolixin Injection**, or *Fluphenazine Decanoate*) 100
Prolongatum (**Mellaril**, or *Thioridazine*) 100
Proma (**Sparine**, or *Promazine*) 100
Promactil (**Sparine**, or *Promazine*) 100
Promapar (**Sparine**, or *Promazine*) 100
Promazil (**Sparine**, or *Promazine*) 100
Promazin (**Sparine**, or *Promazine*) 100
Promazina (**Sparine**, or *Promazine*) 100
Promazine (**Sparine**) 100
Promiben (**Tofranil**, or *Imipramine*) 43
Promwill (**Sparine**, or *Promazine*) 100
Pronoran (**Trivastal**, or *Piribedil*) 59
Propaphenin (**Sparine**, or *Promazine*) 100
Properidol (**Inapsine**, or *Droperidol*) 102
2-propyl-Pentanoic acid (**Depakene**, or *Valproic Acid*) 75
2-propyl-Valeric acid (**Depakene**, or *Valproic Acid*) 75
Propylvaleric acid (**Depakote**, or *Divalproex*) 75
Prostaglandin E1 (**Muse**, or *Alprostadil*) 114
Prostigmin (*Neostigmine*) 123
Prostin VR (**Muse**, or *Alprostadil*) 114
Prostin VR Pediatric (**Muse**, or *Alprostadil*) 114

Rivotril (**Klonopin**, or *Clonazepam*) 83

Romtiazin (**Sparine**, or *Promazine*) 100

Ronyl (**Cylert**, or *Pemoline*) 63

Ropinirol (**Requip**, or *Ropinirole*) 59

Ropinirole (**Requip**) 59

Ropinirolum (**Requip**, or *Ropinirole*) 59

Rowexetina (**Prozac**, or *Fluoxetine*) 47

Ruhsitus (**Valium**, or *Diazepam*) 83

Rulivan (**Serzone**, or *Nefazodone*) 49

S-adenosylmethionine (**SAM-e**) 32

S.A. R.L. (**Valium**, or *Diazepam*) 83

Saint John's Wort (**St. John's Wort**, or *Hypericum*) 30

SAM-e (*S-adenosylmethionine*) 32

Sanopron (**Sparine**, or *Promazine*) 100

Sanzur (**Prozac**, or *Fluoxetine*) 47

Sapilent (**Surmontil**, or *Trimipramine*) 43

Sarafem (**Prozac**, or *Fluoxetine*) 47

Saromet (**Valium**, or *Diazepam*) 83

Saroten (**Elavil**, or *Amitriptyline*) 43

Sarotex (**Elavil**, or *Amitriptyline*) 43

Sd Deprenyl (**Eldepryl**, or *Selegiline (oral)*) 37

Securit (**Ativan**, or *Lorazepam*) 83

Sedacoroxen (**Tofranil**, or *Imipramine*) 43

Sedapam (**Valium**, or *Diazepam*) 83

Sedatival (**Ativan**, or *Lorazepam*) 83

Sedazin (**Ativan**, or *Lorazepam*) 83

Sedipam (**Valium**, or *Diazepam*) 83

Seduksen (**Valium**, or *Diazepam*) 83

Seduxen (**Valium**, or *Diazepam*) 83

Selegeline Hcl (**Eldepryl**, or *Selegiline (oral)*) 37

Selegilina (**Eldepryl**, or *Selegiline (oral)*) 37

Selegiline (oral) (**Eldepryl**) 37

Selegiline (patch) (**Emsam**) 37

Selegiline-5 (**Eldepryl**, or *Selegiline (oral)*) 37

Selegilinum (**Eldepryl**, or *Selegiline (oral)*) 37

Selpak (**Eldepryl**, or *Selegiline (oral)*) 37

Senior (**Cylert**, or *Pemoline*) 63

Sensaval (**Pamelor**, or *Nortriptyline*) 43

Sensival Ventyl (**Pamelor**, or *Nortriptyline*) 43

Sequinan (**Risperdal**, or *Risperidone*) 108

Serdolect (*Sertindole*) 108

Serenace (**Haldol**, or *Haloperidol*) 101

Serenack (**Valium**, or *Diazepam*) 83

Serenamin (**Valium**, or *Diazepam*) 83
Serenase (**Haldol**, or *Haloperidol*) 101
Serenelfi (**Haldol**, or *Haloperidol*) 101
Serentil (*Mesoridazine*) 100
Serenzin (**Valium**, or *Diazepam*) 83
Sernas (**Haldol**, or *Haloperidol*) 101
Sernel (**Haldol**, or *Haloperidol*) 101
Sernevin (**Dolmatil**, or *Sulpiride*) 108
Seropram (**Celexa**, or *Citalopram*) 47
Seroquel (*Quetiapine*) 108
Seroten (**Elavil**, or *Amitriptyline*) 43
Seroxat (**Paxil**, or *Paroxetine*) 47
Sertindole (**Serdolect**) 108
Sertofran (**Norpramin**, or *Desipramine*) 43
Sertofren (**Norpramin**, or *Desipramine*) 43
Sertralina (**Zoloft**, or *Sertraline*) 47
Sertraline (**Zoloft**) 47
Sertralinum (**Zoloft**, or *Sertraline*) 47
Servizepam (**Valium**, or *Diazepam*) 83
Servox (**Luvox**, or *Fluvoxamine*) 47
Serzone (*Nefazodone*) 49
Sesaval (**Pamelor**, or *Nortriptyline*) 43
Setonil (**Valium**, or *Diazepam*) 83
Sevinol (**Prolixin Injection**, or *Fluphenazine Decanoate*) 100
Sibazon (**Valium**, or *Diazepam*) 83
Sibazone (**Valium**, or *Diazepam*) 83
Sicoton (**Parnate**, or *Tranylcypromine*) 39
Sideril (**Desyrel**, or *Trazodone*) 49
Sigaperidol (**Haldol**, or *Haloperidol*) 101
Sigmadyn (**Cylert**, or *Pemoline*) 63
Sildenafil (**Viagra**) 114
Silibrin (**Librium**, or *Chlordiazepoxide*) 83
Simpatedrin (**Dexedrine**, or *Dextroamphetamine*) 63
Simpatina (**Dexedrine**, or *Dextroamphetamine*) 63
Sinequan (*Doxepin*) 43
Sinophenin (**Sparine**, or *Promazine*) 100
Sintodril (**Inapsine**, or *Droperidol*) 102
Sintosian (**Inapsine**, or *Droperidol*) 102
Siplaril (**Depixol**, or *Flupenthixol*) 101
Siplarol (**Depixol**, or *Flupenthixol*) 101
Siqualine (**Prolixin Injection**, or *Fluphenazine Decanoate*) 100
Siqualon (**Prolixin Injection**, or *Fluphenazine Decanoate*) 100
Sirtal (**Tegretol**, or *Carbamazepine*) 77

Sursumid (**Dolmatil**, or *Sulpiride*) 108
Survector (*Amineptine*) 56
Sylvemid (**Elavil**, or *Amitriptyline*) 43
Symadine (**Symmetrel**, or *Amantadine*) 59
Symbyax (*Fluoxetine + Olanzapine*) 47
Symmetrel (*Amantadine*) 59
Sympamin (**Dexedrine**, or *Dextroamphetamine*) 63
Sympamine (**Dexedrine**, or *Dextroamphetamine*) 63
Sympatedrine (**Dexedrine**, or *Dextroamphetamine*) 63
Synedil (**Dolmatil**, or *Sulpiride*) 108
Synklor (**Stelazine**, or *Trifluoperazine*) 100
Tactaran (**Truxal**, or *Chlorprothixene*) 101
Tadalafil (**Cialis**) 114
Tadanafil (**Cialis**, or *Tadalafil*) 114
Tafil (**Xanax**, or *Alprazolam*) 83
Taractan (**Truxal**, or *Chlorprothixene*) 101
Tarasan (**Truxal**, or *Chlorprothixene*) 101
Tardan (**Truxal**, or *Chlorprothixene*) 101
Tardotol (**Tegretol**, or *Carbamazepine*) 77
Taro-Carbamazepine (**Tegretol**, or *Carbamazepine*) 77
Taro-Carbamazepine Cr (**Tegretol**, or *Carbamazepine*) 77
Taver (**Tegretol**, or *Carbamazepine*) 77
Tavor (**Ativan**, or *Lorazepam*) 83
Taxagon (**Desyrel**, or *Trazodone*) 49
Tegol (**Tegretol**, or *Carbamazepine*) 77
Tegretal (**Tegretol**, or *Carbamazepine*) 77
Tegretol (*Carbamazepine*) 77
Tegretol Chewtabs (**Tegretol**, or *Carbamazepine*) 77
Tegretol Cr (**Tegretol**, or *Carbamazepine*) 77
Tegretol-Xr (**Tegretol**, or *Carbamazepine*) 77
Telesmin (**Tegretol**, or *Carbamazepine*) 77
Telestin (**Tegretol**, or *Carbamazepine*) 77
Tementil (**Compazine**, or *Prochlorperazine*) 100
Temesta (**Ativan**, or *Lorazepam*) 83
Temetid (**Compazine**, or *Prochlorperazine*) 100
Temporal Slow (**Tegretol**, or *Carbamazepine*) 77
Temporol (**Tegretol**, or *Carbamazepine*) 77
Tensofin (**Prolixin Injection**, or *Fluphenazine Decanoate*) 100
Tensopam (**Valium**, or *Diazepam*) 83
Teralithe (**Lithobid**, or *Lithium Carbonate*) 73
Terfluzine (**Stelazine**, or *Trifluoperazine*) 100
Teril (**Tegretol**, or *Carbamazepine*) 77
Thaden (**Prothiaden**, or *Dothiepin*) 43

Tradone (**Cylert**, or *Pemoline*) 63

Tranax (**Xanax**, or *Alprazolam*) 83

Tranimul (**Valium**, or *Diazepam*) 83

Trankimazin (**Xanax**, or *Alprazolam*) 83

Tranqdyn (**Valium**, or *Diazepam*) 83

Tranquase (**Valium**, or *Diazepam*) 83

Tranquilan (**Truxal**, or *Chlorprothixene*) 101

Tranquinal (**Xanax**, or *Alprazolam*) 83

Tranquirit (**Valium**, or *Diazepam*) 83

Tranquisan (**Trilafon**, or *Perphenazine*) 100

Tranquo-Puren (**Valium**, or *Diazepam*) 83

Tranquo-Tablinen (**Valium**, or *Diazepam*) 83

Transamin (**Parnate**, or *Tranylcypromine*) 39

Transamine (**Parnate**, or *Tranylcypromine*) 39

Transapin (**Parnate**, or *Tranylcypromine*) 39

Tranxene (*Clorazepate*) 83

Tranylcypromine (**Parnate**) 39

Traquilan (**Truxal**, or *Chlorprothixene*) 101

Travin (**BuSpar**, or *Buspirone*) 119

Trazalon (**Desyrel**, or *Trazodone*) 49

Trazine (**Stelazine**, or *Trifluoperazine*) 100

Trazodil (**Desyrel**, or *Trazodone*) 49

Trazodon (**Desyrel**, or *Trazodone*) 49

Trazodona (**Desyrel**, or *Trazodone*) 49

Trazodone (**Desyrel**) 49

Trazodonum (**Desyrel**, or *Trazodone*) 49

Trazolan (**Desyrel**, or *Trazodone*) 49

Trazonil (**Desyrel**, or *Trazodone*) 49

Trevilor (**Effexor**, or *Venlafaxine*) 50

Triadapin (**Sinequan**, or *Doxepin*) 43

Triadapin 5 (**Vivactil**, or *Protriptyline*) 43

Trialodine (**Desyrel**, or *Trazodone*) 49

Triavil (**Trilafon**, or *Perphenazine*) 100

Trictal (**Truxal**, or *Chlorprothixene*) 101

Tridep (**Elavil**, or *Amitriptyline*) 43

Trifaron (**Trilafon**, or *Perphenazine*) 100

Triflumethazine (**Prolixin Injection**, or *Fluphenazine Decanoate*) 100

Trifluoperazine (**Stelazine**) 100

Trifluoperazin (**Stelazine**, or *Trifluoperazine*) 100

Trifluoperazina (**Stelazine**, or *Trifluoperazine*) 100

Trifluoromethylperazine (**Stelazine**, or *Trifluoperazine*) 100

Trifluoroperazine (**Stelazine**, or *Trifluoperazine*) 100

Trifluperazine (**Stelazine**, or *Trifluoperazine*) 100

Urecholine (*Bethanechol*) 123
Urecholine Chloride (**Urecholine**, or *Bethanechol*) 123
Uro-Carb (**Urecholine**, or *Bethanechol*) 123
Usaf Sz-3 (**Mellaril**, or *Thioridazine*) 100
Usaf Sz-B (**Mellaril**, or *Thioridazine*) 100
Usempax Ap (**Valium**, or *Diazepam*) 83
Uxen (**Elavil**, or *Amitriptyline*) 43
Valamina (**Prolixin Injection**, or *Fluphenazine Decanoate*) 100
Valaxona (**Valium**, or *Diazepam*) 83
Valcote (**Depakote**, or *Divalproex*) 75
Valeo (**Valium**, or *Diazepam*) 83
Valeptol (**Depacon**, or *Sodium Valproate*) 75
Valiquid (**Valium**, or *Diazepam*) 83
Valirem (**Dolmatil**, or *Sulpiride*) 108
Valitran (**Valium**, or *Diazepam*) 83
Valium (*Diazepam*) 83
Valnar (**Depakote**, or *Divalproex*) 75
Valoin (**Depacon**, or *Sodium Valproate*) 75
Valpakine (**Depacon**, or *Sodium Valproate*) 75
Valparin (**Depacon**, or *Sodium Valproate*) 75
Valporal (**Depacon**, or *Sodium Valproate*) 75
Valprax (**Depacon**, or *Sodium Valproate*) 75
Valpro (**Depacon**, or *Sodium Valproate*) 75
Valproate semisodique (**Depakene**, or *Valproic Acid*) 75
Valproate semisodium (**Depakene**, or *Valproic Acid*) 75
Valproato semisodico (**Depakene**, or *Valproic Acid*) 75
Valproatum seminatricum (**Depakene**, or *Valproic Acid*) 75
Valproic Acid (**Depakene**) 75
Valprosid (**Depakene**, or *Valproic Acid*) 75
Valrelease (**Valium**, or *Diazepam*) 83
Valsup (**Depacon**, or *Sodium Valproate*) 75
Vanatrip (**Elavil**, or *Amitriptyline*) 43
Vandral (**Effexor**, or *Venlafaxine*) 50
Vardenafil (**Levitra**) 114
Vatran (**Valium**, or *Diazepam*) 83
VDN (**Levitra**, or *Vardenafil*) 114
Velium (**Valium**, or *Diazepam*) 83
Venefon (**Tofranil**, or *Imipramine*) 43
Venlafaxine (**Effexor**) 50
Venlafaxina (**Effexor**, or *Venlafaxine*) 50
Verophen (**Sparine**, or *Promazine*) 100
Vertigon (**Compazine**, or *Prochlorperazine*) 100
Vesalium (**Haldol**, or *Haloperidol*) 101

Vespazine (**Prolixin Injection**, or *Fluphenazine Decanoate*) 100
Vesprin (**Sparine**, or *Promazine*) 100
Vestra (**Edronax**, or *Reboxetine*) 52
Vetacalm (**Truxal**, or *Chlorprothixene*) 101
Vetkalm (**Inapsine**, or *Droperidol*) 102
Viagra (*Sildenafil*) 114
Vikonon (**Yocon**, or *Yohimbine*) 116
Viopsicol (**Librium**, or *Chlordiazepoxide*) 83
Vivactil (*Protriptyline*) 43
Vival (**Valium**, or *Diazepam*) 83
Vividyl (**Pamelor**, or *Nortriptyline*) 43
Vivol (**Valium**, or *Diazepam*) 83
Volital (**Cylert**, or *Pemoline*) 63
Volitol (**Cylert**, or *Pemoline*) 63
Vyvanse (*Lisdexamfetamine*) 63
Weckamine (**Dexedrine**, or *Dextroamphetamine*) 63
Wellbatrin (**Wellbutrin**, or *Bupropion*) 53
Wellbutrin (*Bupropion*) 53
Wintermin (**Sparine**, or *Promazine*) 100
Wypax (**Ativan**, or *Lorazepam*) 83
Xanax (*Alprazolam*) 83
Xanax XR (**Xanax**, or *Alprazolam*) 83
Xanor (**Xanax**, or *Alprazolam*) 83
Yentreve (**Cymbalta**, or *Duloxetine*) 50
Yespazine (**Prolixin Injection**, or *Fluphenazine Decanoate*) 100
Yh 1 (**Cylert**, or *Pemoline*) 63
Yocon (*Yohimbine*) 116
Yohimbine (**Yocon**) 116
Yohimex (**Yocon**, or *Yohimbine*) 116
Yohydrol (**Yocon**, or *Yohimbine*) 116
Zactin (**Prozac**, or *Fluoxetine*) 47
Zelapar (**Eldepryl**, or *Selegiline (oral)*) 37
Zeldox (**Geodon**, or *Ziprasidone*) 108
Zemorcon (**Dolmatil**, or *Sulpiride*) 108
Zepax. (**Prozac**, or *Fluoxetine*) 47
Zetran (**Valium**, or *Diazepam*) 83
Zipan (**Valium**, or *Diazepam*) 83
Ziprasidone (**Geodon**) 108
Zispin (**Remeron**, or *Mirtazapine*) 54
Zoleptil (*Zotepine*) 108
Zoloft (*Sertraline*) 47
Zonalon (**Sinequan**, or *Doxepin*) 43
Zotepine (**Zoleptil**) 108

About the Author

Kevin Thompson, Ph.D., is a physicist who has an interest in medical treatments for mental illness. He received his doctorate in physics from Princeton University in 1985, and has worked for NASA and a variety of high-technology companies since then. Dr. Thompson has written technical articles and books in areas such as computational fluid dynamics, relativistic astrophysics, and computer languages. *Medicines for Mental Health* is his first book for the general public, and his first in the field of medical science.

3120599

Made in the USA